# Unbelievable Paleo

**A Paleo Cookbook to Lose Weight and Reboot Your Health**

**Jamie Evans**

# © Copyright 2021 - All rights reserved.

# TABLE OF CONTENTS

---- DINNER ----

## ---- DESSERTS ----

## ---- SNACKS ----

# Breakfast

# ROOT VEGETABLE OMELET

This easy to prepare omelet is loaded with root veggies, for fiber and antioxidants.

MAKES 1 SERVING/ TOTAL TIME 5 MINUTE

## INGREDIENTS

1 tablespoon olive oil

1/2 cup grated root vegetables such as beets, turnips, or parsnips

3 eggs beaten

1 ounce goat cheese crumbled

1 tablespoon fresh chopped parsley

Sea salt and fresh ground pepper to taste

## METHOD

### STEP 1

In a non-stick skillet, heat the oil over medium heat. Add the root veggies and cook until softened and lightly caramelized. Season with salt and pepper and add the eggs. Cook for a minute until the edges are set.

### STEP 2

Lift the edges carefully and let the liquid flow underneath the edges. When eggs are cooked, top with the goat cheese crumbles. Cover until warmed through and serve.

**NUTRITION  VALUE**

500 Kcal, 20g fat,
14g fiber, 24g protein, 14g carbs.

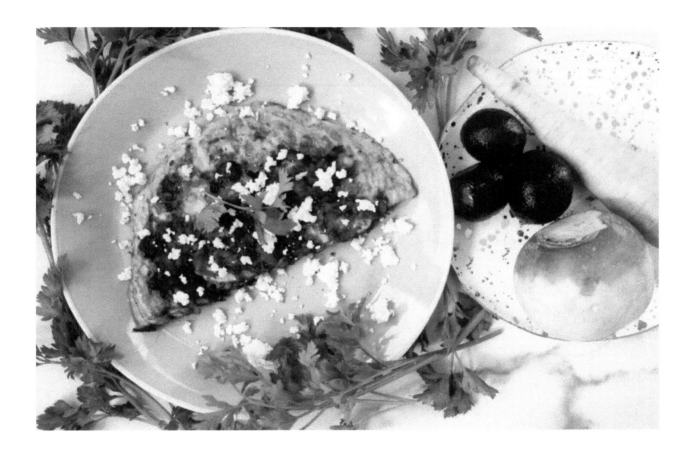

# BRUSSELS SPROUT HASH WITH FRIED EGGS

Bacon and shredded Brussels sprouts are the perfect flavorful accompaniment to your fried eggs for breakfast.

MAKES 2 SERVING/ TOTAL TIME 20 MINUTE

## INGREDIENTS

4 slices bacon diced

1 onion chopped

2 cloves garlic minced

3 cups cored and shredded Brussels sprouts

1 teaspoon lemon pepper seasoning

1 tablespoon olive oil

4 eggs

Sea salt and fresh ground pepper to taste

## METHOD

STEP 1

In a heavy nonstick skillet, cook the bacon until crisp. Remove with a slotted spoon and drain paper towels. Add the onion to the pan and cook until softened. Add the garlic and cook for about 30 seconds.

**STEP 2**

Stir in the Brussels sprouts and lemon pepper seasoning, and stir and cook until softened and lightly browned. Remove from pan.
Add the olive oil and crack the eggs in the pan. Fry to your liking.
Serve the eggs over top the hash.

**NUTRITION  VALUE**

447 Kcal, 20g fat,
5g fiber, 21g protein, 14.6g carbs.

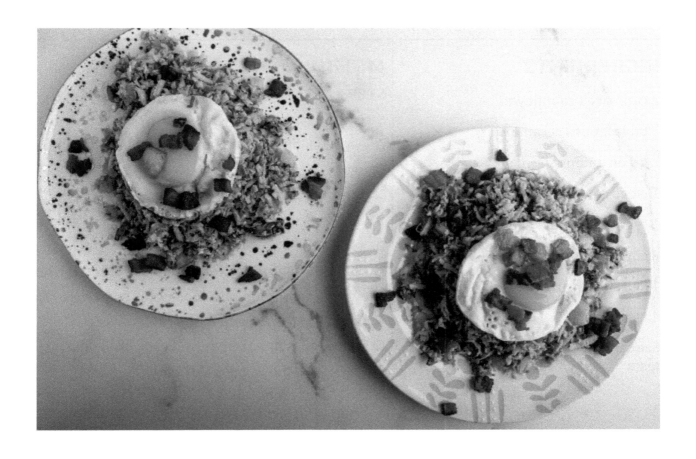

# BREAKFAST STIR-FRY

This easy to make breakfast is a different take on the usual omelet or pancakes. It's full of fiber and protein, and is sure to keep you full all day long.

MAKES 2 SERVING/ TOTAL TIME 20 MINUTE

## INGREDIENTS

2 cups riced cauliflower

2 tablespoons sesame oil

2 green onions sliced

1 clove garlic minced

1 teaspoon grated ginger

2 cups chopped bok choy or cabbage

1 cup sliced carrots

4 eggs

Sea salt and fresh ground pepper to taste

## METHOD

### STEP 1

Steam the cauliflower in the microwave until tender. Add a pinch of salt and pepper. Divide between two plates.

### STEP 2

In a large skillet, heat the oil and add the green onions, garlic, and ginger. Cook for a minute and add the bok choy and carrots. Stir and cook until veggies are crisp tender. Remove and add to the cauliflower.
Crack the eggs into the pan and cook until done to your liking. Add to the veggies and serve.

**NUTRITION  VALUE**

331 Kcal, 20g fat,
5g fiber, 22g protein, 13g carbs.

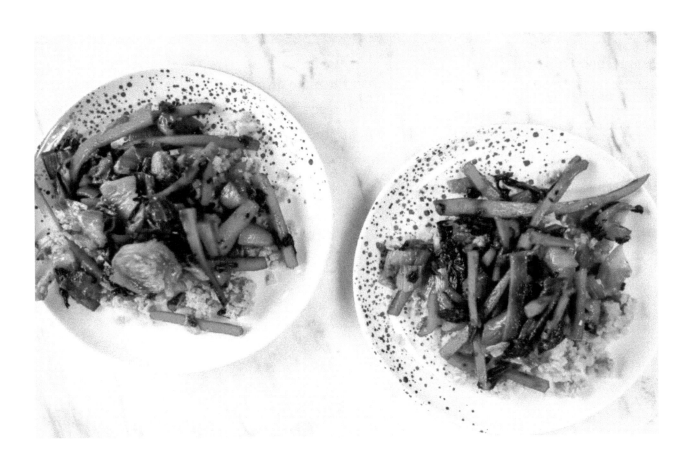

# GREEK OMELET

Salty olives and sundried tomatoes takes the omelet a long way when it comes to flavor and nutrition. This is the perfect breakfast when you're short on time but still need a healthy breakfast.

MAKES 1 SERVING/ TOTAL TIME 10 MINUTE

## INGREDIENTS

1 tablespoon olive oil

3 eggs beaten

1/4 cup diced cucumber

1/4 cup diced red onion

2 tablespoons sliced sundried tomatoes

4-5 kalamata olives pitted and sliced

1/4 teaspoon dried oregano

Sea salt and fresh ground pepper to taste

## METHOD
### STEP 1

Heat the oil in a small skillet over medium low heat. Add the eggs and cook for a minute until the edges are set. Lift the edges carefully and let the liquid flow underneath the edges.

### STEP 2

When the eggs are cooked, add the remaining ingredients and fold in half. Heat through and serve.

| NUTRITION VALUE | 470 Kcal, 20g fat, 3g fiber, 21g protein, 14g carbs. |
|---|---|

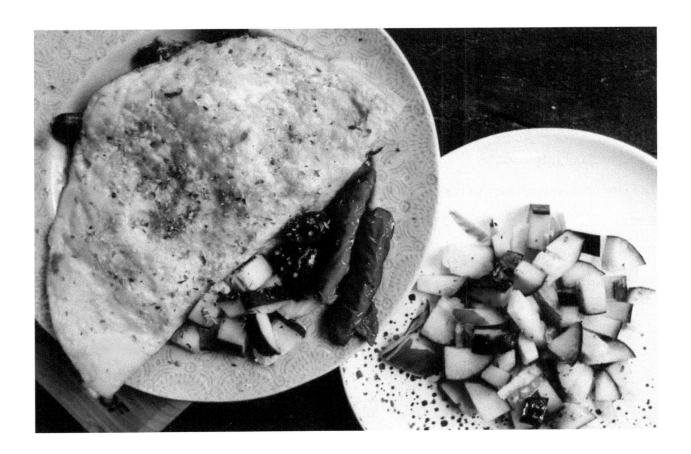

# BREAKFAST NOODLE BOWL

Zucchini noodles are paired with eggs and flavorful broth for a different kind of breakfast that will soon become a favorite.

MAKES 2 SERVING/ TOTAL TIME 20 MINUTE

## INGREDIENTS

1 tablespoon olive oil

1 onion sliced

2 cloves garlic minced

1 teaspoon grated ginger

2 zucchini cut into noodles

1/2 cup homemade chicken broth

4 eggs

1 teaspoon vinegar

Sea salt and fresh ground pepper to taste

## METHOD

### STEP 1

Heat the oil in a large skillet over medium heat and add the onion, garlic, and ginger. Cook until softened and add the zucchini noodles. Stir and cook for about 2 minutes and add the broth.

### STEP 2

Before serving, crack the eggs in a small bowl one at a time. Bring a pan of water to a simmer and add the vinegar. Carefully add the eggs and turn off the heat. Cook for 4 minutes. Remove with a slotted spoon and serve on top of the vegetables.

**NUTRITION  VALUE**

332 Kcal, 8.7g fat, 13.6g fiber, 21g protein, 14g carbs.

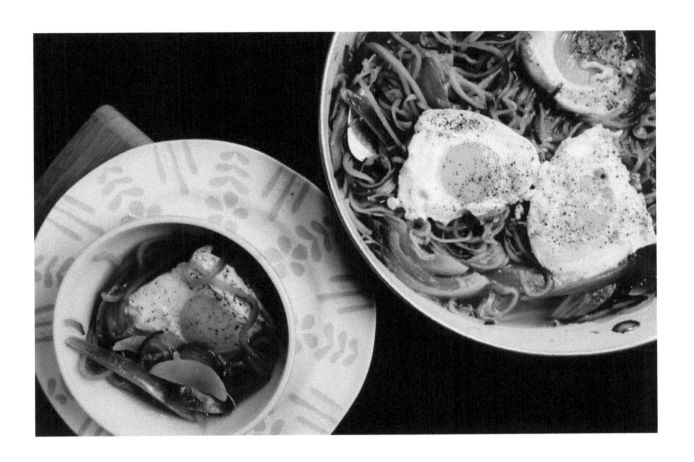

# SOUTHWEST TURKEY HASH

Never discount the amount of flavor you can get from a simple combo of spices. Some ground turkey and sweet potatoes provide a filling, nutritionally sound breakfast on a busy day.

MAKES 2 SERVING/ TOTAL TIME 25 MINUTE

## INGREDIENTS

1 tablespoon olive oil

1 onion diced

1 bell pepper diced

1 sweet potato peeled and diced

1/2 teaspoon chili powder

1/2 teaspoon oregano

1/2 teaspoon cumin

1/2-pound ground turkey

4 eggs

Sea salt and fresh ground pepper to taste

## METHOD

**STEP 1**

Heat the oil over medium high heat. Add the onion, pepper, and sweet potatoes. Cook until veggies are softened. Add the seasonings and cook for another minute.

**STEP 2**

Add the turkey to the pan and stir and cook until turkey is cooked through.

Using a spatula, form 4 small holes in the hash and crack the eggs inside. Cook until eggs are done to your liking and serve.

**NUTRITION VALUE**

493 Kcal, 20g fat,
6g fiber, 38g protein, 14.8g carbs.

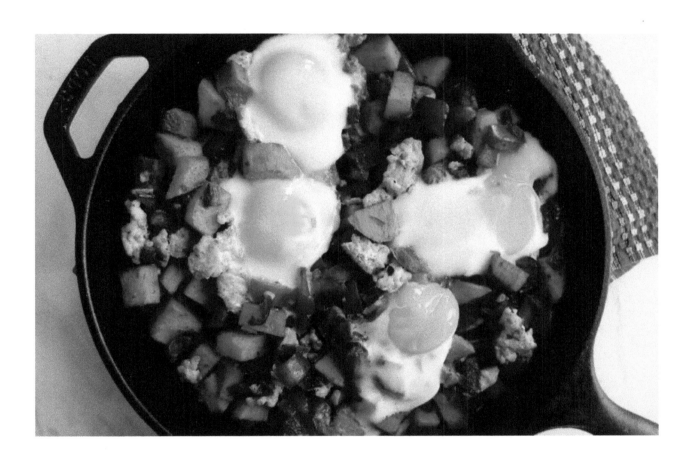

# Lunch

# PESTO SHRIMP SALAD

This easy shrimp salad comes together quickly and tastes amazing. Perfect for a quick lunch that is high in protein and flavor.

MAKES 1 SERVING/ TOTAL TIME 10 MINUTE

## INGREDIENTS

1/2 cup basil leaves

1 clove garlic

2 tablespoons chopped walnuts

Juice of 1 lemon

1/4 cup olive oil

2 5- ounce cans cooked shrimp drained

1 cup halved cherry tomatoes

1 small red onion sliced

2 cups arugula

Sea salt and fresh ground pepper to taste

## METHOD

### STEP 1

Put the basil, garlic, walnuts, lemon juice, and olive oil in blender or food processor and blend until smooth. Toss the pesto with the remaining ingredients, and chill until ready to serve.

| NUTRITION VALUE | 410 Kcal, 20g fat, 4g fiber, 26g protein, 11g carbs. |
|---|---|

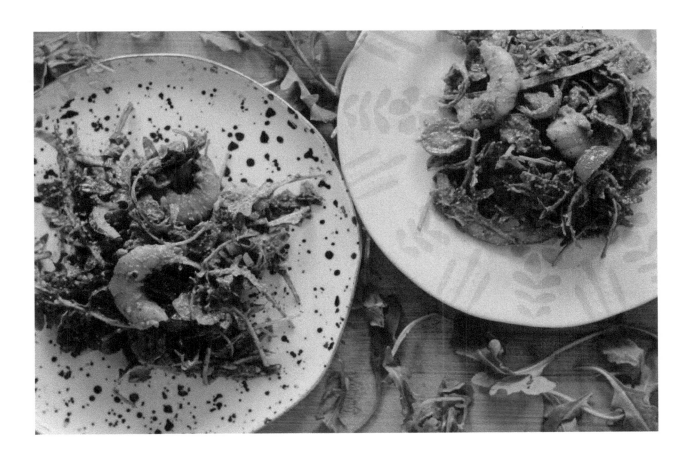

# BALSAMIC GRILLED PORK TENDERLOIN

Instead of grilling the same chicken breast or burgers, try your hand at this easy balsamic pork tenderloin. It's juicy and flavorful, and perfect with your favorite vegetable or salad.

MAKES 4 SERVING/ TOTAL TIME 40 MINUTE

## INGREDIENTS

1/2 cup balsamic vinegar

2 tablespoons honey

1 teaspoon crushed red pepper flakes

1/2 teaspoon sea salt

1/2 teaspoon black pepper

1 pork tenderloin

## METHOD

### STEP 1

Put all of the ingredients in a freezer bag and mix well, covering the pork. Marinate in the refrigerator for 1-2 hours.

### STEP 2

When ready to cook, preheat grill to medium high heat. Grill the pork until internal temperature reaches 165 degrees F. Let rest for 10-15 minutes before slicing. Serve with your favorite vegetables on the side.

## NUTRITION VALUE

353 Kcal, 10g fat, 58g protein, 14g carbs.

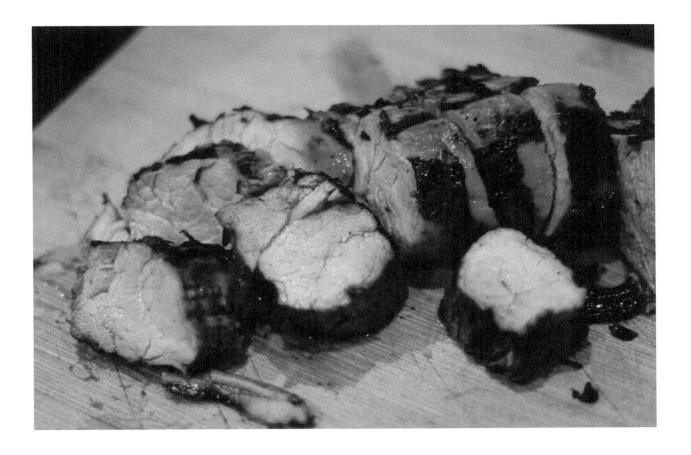

# TUNA CAKES WITH LEMON PARSLEY SLAW

Turn a can of tuna into an easy and nutritious meal with this easy recipe. It's perfect for a quick lunch or dinner, and makes a filling meal you can count on.

MAKES 2 SERVING/ TOTAL TIME 20 MINUTE

## INGREDIENTS

Lemon Parsley Slaw:

2 tablespoons olive oil-based mayonnaise

Juice and zest of 1/2 lemon

1 clove garlic minced

2 tablespoons finely chopped parsley

2 cups finely shredded cabbage

Sea salt and fresh ground pepper to taste

Tuna Cakes:

2 5- ounce cans tuna drained

4 green onions sliced

1 clove garlic minced

Juice and zest of 1/2 lemon

1/2 cup almond flour

1/2 teaspoon sea salt

2 eggs

## METHOD

### STEP 1

Make the slaw by whisking the mayo, lemon, and garlic in a large bowl. Add the cabbage and parsley, season with salt and pepper. Stir and set aside.

### STEP 2

To make the tuna cakes, mix the tuna, green onions, garlic, lemon, almond flour, salt and eggs in a large bowl. Mix well and form into 4 patties.
Heat a skillet over medium high heat and add the oil. Fry the tuna cakes until browned on both sides. Serve over the slaw.

| NUTRITION VALUE | 351 Kcal, 20g fat, 5g fiber, 22g protein, 10g carbs. |
|---|---|

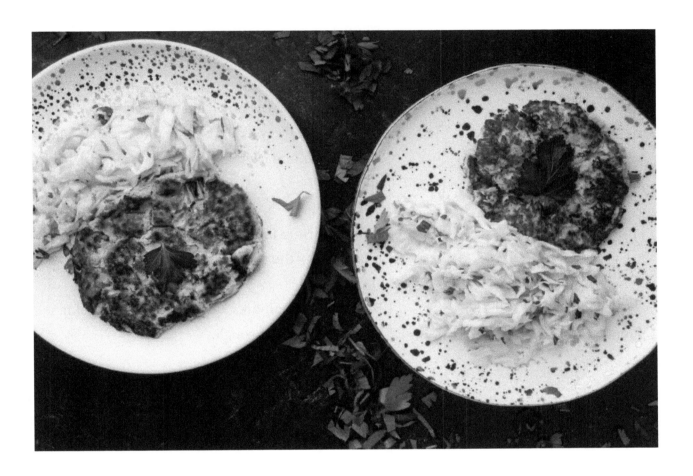

# COCONUT SHRIMP WITH MANGO SLAW

A sweet and savory salad is served with crispy coconut shrimp for a meal that is nutritious, filling, and satisfying.

MAKES 2 SERVING/ TOTAL TIME 20 MINUTE

## INGREDIENTS

2 cups finely shredded cabbage

1 jalapeno minced

1 mango diced

1/2 cup chopped cilantro

Juice of 1 lime

1/2 cup unsweetened shredded coconut

1/2 cup almond flour

1/2 teaspoon garlic powder

1/4 teaspoon cayenne pepper

1 pound peeled and deveined shrimp

1 egg

## METHOD

**STEP 1**

Preheat oven to 400 degrees F.

Combine the cabbage, jalapeno, mango cilantro, and lime juice in a large bowl and toss. Set aside.

In a wide, shallow dish, combine the coconut, almond flour, garlic, and cayenne. In a separate bowl, beat the egg.

**STEP 2**

Dip the shrimp in the egg, followed by the coconut mixture. Lay the shrimp on a parchment lined baking sheet.

Bake for 8-10 minutes, until the shrimp is golden brown and cook through.

Serve with the slaw.

**NUTRITION VALUE**

469 Kcal, 19g fat,
8g fiber, 45g protein, 15g carbs.

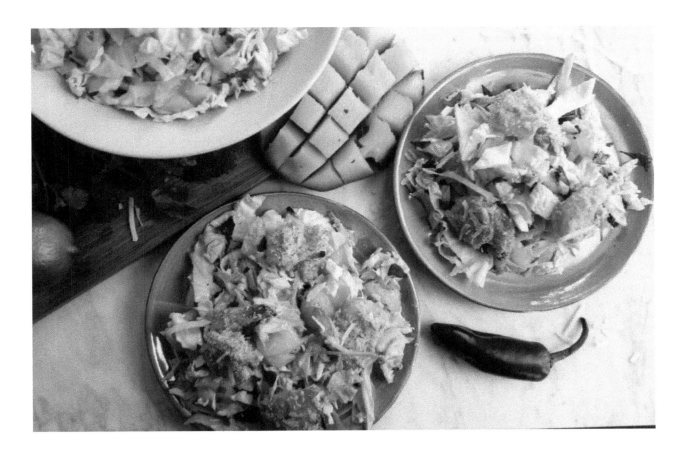

# LEMON CAPER CHICKEN AND GARLIC SPINACH

Capers add a ton of flavor to this dish without any bad stuff, and when paired with garlicky spinach, this becomes an amazing meal.

MAKES 2 SERVING/ TOTAL TIME 30 MINUTE

## INGREDIENTS

2 chicken breasts

2 tablespoons olive oil

Juice of 1 lemon

2 tablespoons capers

2 cloves garlic minced

6 cups baby spinach

Sea salt and fresh ground pepper to taste

## METHOD

### STEP 1

Using a meat mallet, pound the chicken breasts until they are an even thickness. Season with salt and pepper.

Heat half the oil over medium high heat in a heavy skillet and add the chicken. Cook until chicken easily releases from the pan with a spatula and flip. Add the lemon juice and capers to the pan.

### STEP 2

Cover and cook on low for 5 minutes.

Remove chicken from the pan, and add the remaining oil. Add the garlic and sauté for 30 seconds. Add the spinach to the pan as quickly as you can and cook until wilted.

Serve the spinach with the chicken.

| NUTRITION VALUE | 256 Kcal, 15g fat, 3g fiber, 23g protein, 8g carbs. |
|---|---|

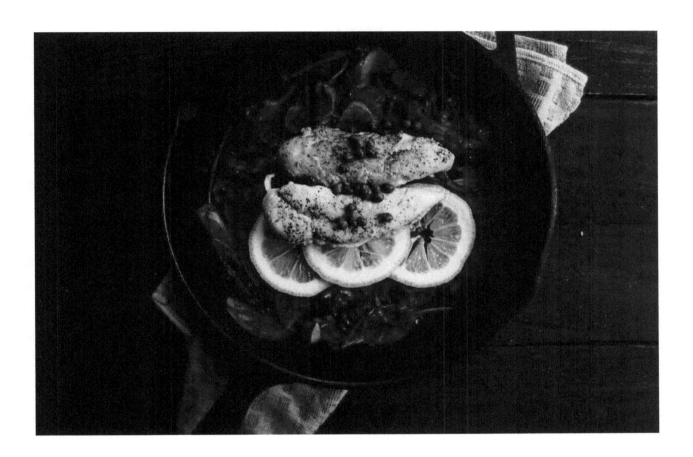

# CASHEW ORANGE CHICKEN

For the perfect combination of sweet and salty, this dish has it all — healthy protein, heart healthy fats, and lots of vitamins and minerals.

MAKES 4 SERVING/ TOTAL TIME 45 MINUTE

## INGREDIENTS

2 cup pineapple juice

Juice and zest of 2 oranges

2 tablespoons coconut sugar

1 tablespoon Paleo fish sauce

1 1/2 pounds chicken breast cut into bite sized pieces

1/2 cup almond flour

4 cups cauliflower rice

4 green onions sliced

1/2 cup roasted cashews

Sea salt and fresh ground pepper to taste

## METHOD

### STEP 1

Preheat oven to 400 degrees F. Line a baking sheet with parchment paper or foil.

Put the pineapple juice, orange juice and zest, coconut sugar, and fish sauce in a large saucepan. Bring to a boil and reduce to a low simmer. Simmer for 15 minutes, until reduced to a thick syrup. Remove from heat. Add the chicken pieces and coat well.

### STEP 2

Dredge the coated chicken pieces with the almond flour and transfer to baking sheet. Bake for 10-15 minutes, until chicken is cooked through.

While the chicken is baking, steam the cauliflower rice with the green onions until tender and then stir in the cashews.

Top the cauliflower rice with the chicken and serve.

| NUTRITION VALUE | 410 Kcal, 12g fat, 3g fiber, 20g protein, 14g carbs. |
| --- | --- |

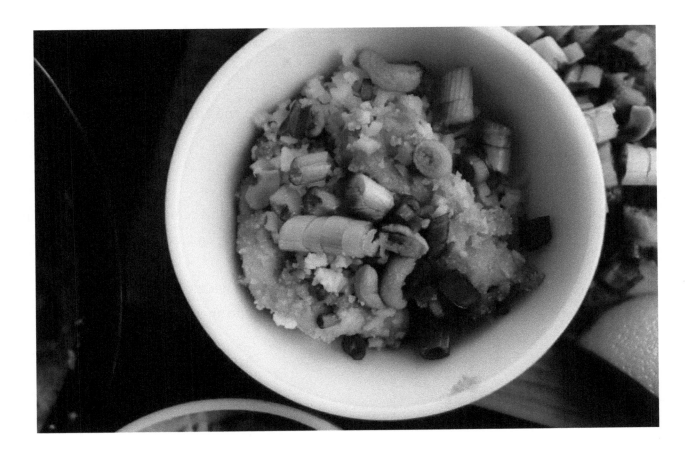

# EGG SALAD STUFFED AVOCADO

Healthy protein and high-quality fats make the perfect lunch. It's also super portable — pack your egg salad and avocado and then assemble right when you're ready to eat.

MAKES 1 SERVING/ TOTAL TIME 15 MINUTE

## INGREDIENTS

2 hard boiled eggs

1 tablespoon Paleo mayonnaise

1 tablespoon relish

1 teaspoon Dijon mustard

1 avocado

Sea salt and fresh ground pepper to taste

## METHOD

### STEP 1

Rough chop the eggs and add to a bowl with the relish, mayo, and mustard.

### STEP 2

Cut the avocado in half and remove the pit. Scoop half the flesh out of each side and add to the bowl with the eggs.

Mash well, and season with salt and pepper.

Spoon into the avocado shells and serve.

**NUTRITION VALUE**

480 Kcal, 20g fat, 10g fiber, 20g protein, 14g carbs.

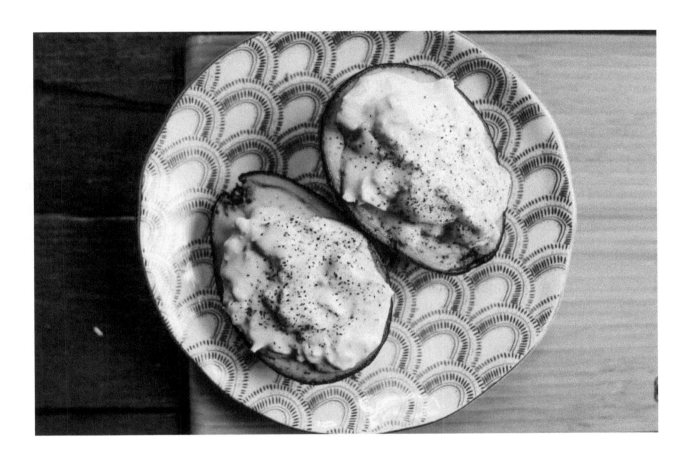

# SALMON KALE SALAD

Pan seared salmon is extra crispy and delicious and adds flavor and protein to this quick and easy salad.

MAKES 2 SERVING/ TOTAL TIME 20 MINUTE

## INGREDIENTS

1/4 cup olive oil plus 1 tablespoon

Juice of 1 lemon

1 clove garlic minced

1 shallot minced

1 teaspoon Dijon mustard

1 bunch of kale shredded

1 cup cherry tomatoes halved

1 small cucumber diced

4 slices cooked and crumbled bacon

2 salmon filets

Sea salt and fresh ground pepper to taste

## METHOD

### STEP 1

Put 1/4 cup olive oil, lemon juice, garlic, shallot, and mustard in a large bowl. Whisk until well combined. Add the kale, tomatoes, and bacon and toss.

### STEP 2

Heat the remaining tablespoon of oil in a heavy skillet. Season the salmon filets with salt and pepper and add to the pan. Cook until golden brown and done to your liking.

Serve on top of the salad.

| NUTRITION VALUE | 531 Kcal, 30g fat, 6g fiber, 29g protein, 15g carbs. |
|---|---|

Unbelievable Paleo   Jamie Evans

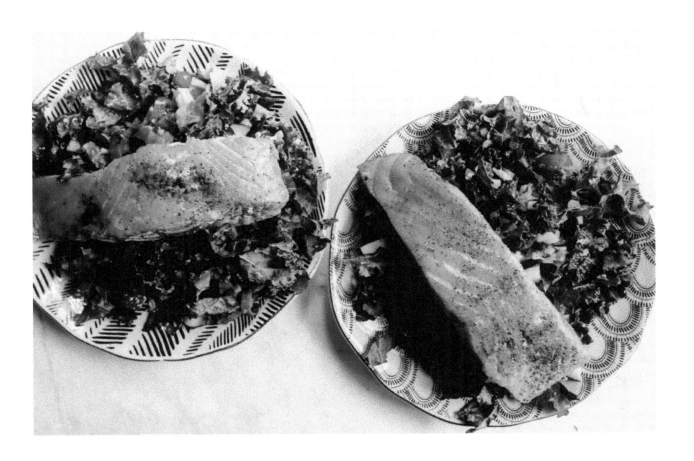

37

# STEAK BURRITO BOWLS

Recipe that Everyone love.

MAKES 2 SERVING/ TOTAL TIME 20 MINUTE

## INGREDIENTS

1 tablespoon olive oil

1/2-pound sirloin steak cut into strips

1 bell pepper sliced

1 onion sliced

1 jalapeno sliced

1 teaspoon chili powder

1 teaspoon cumin

1 teaspoon garlic powder

2 cups riced cauliflower

1/2 cup finely chopped cilantro

Juice of 1 lime

To serve: guacamole salsa, shredded lettuce, hot sauce

## METHOD

### STEP 1

Preheat oven to 450 degrees Toss the oil with the steak, peppers, onions, and seasonings. Lay on a sheet pan and bake for 10-12 minutes, until steak is done and veggies are lightly caramelized. Remove from oven.

### STEP 2

Combine the rice, cilantro, and lime juice in a bowl and steam in the microwave until cauliflower is tender. Season with salt and pepper.

Serve the rice, steak and veggies in a bowl topped with guacamole, salsa, and lettuce.

## NUTRITION VALUE

335 Kcal, 14g fat,
8g fiber, 32g protein, 15g carbs.

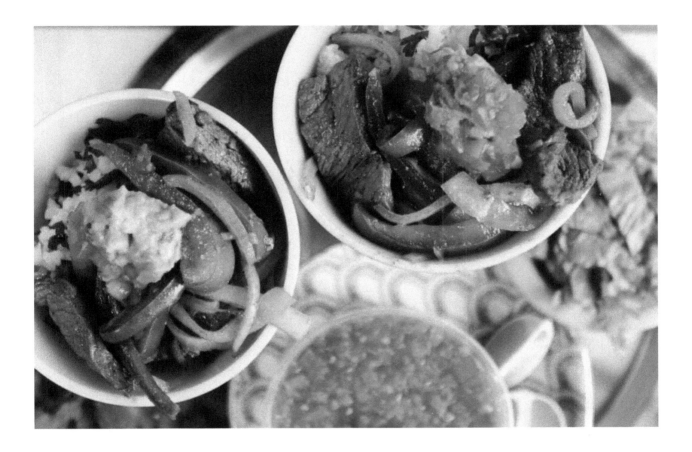

# SHEET PAN CHICKEN FAJITAS

All you have to do is cut your meat up into thin even strips. Cut your veggies up the same way. Throw it all on a pan with some spices and cook for about 15 minutes .

MAKES 4 SERVING/ TOTAL TIME 45 MINUTE

## INGREDIENTS

1.5-pound chicken breast cut into strips

3 bell peppers any color, cut into strips

1 red onion sliced

1 cup sliced mushrooms

1 tsp chili powder

.5 tsp cumin

.5 tsp garlic powder

.5 tsp onion powder

.5 tsp dried oregano

.5 tsp sea salt

.5 cup finely chopped cilantro

juice of 1 lime

large, crisp lettuce leaves

guacamole and salsa for serving

## METHOD
### STEP 1

Preheat oven to 450 degrees F.
Toss the meat, peppers, onions, and mushrooms with the seasonings. Roast for 10-15 minutes until chicken is done and veggies are browned.

### STEP 2
Remove from oven, sprinkle with cilantro and lime juice.
Serve in the lettuce leaves topped with your desired toppings.

## NUTRITION VALUE

335 Kcal, 14g fat,
8g fiber, 32g protein, 15g carbs.

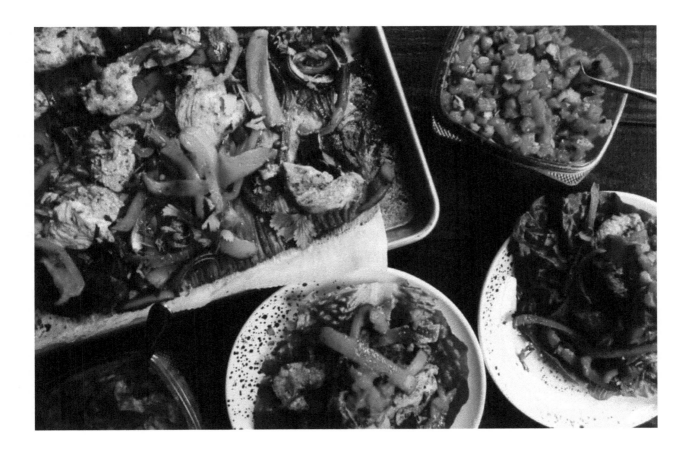

# CURRIED CHICKEN STEW

Recipe that Everyone love.

MAKES 4 SERVING/ TOTAL TIME 30 MINUTE

## INGREDIENTS

4 tablespoons coconut oil

1 onion diced

2 cloves garlic minced

1 teaspoon grated ginger

1 teaspoon curry powder

4 cups chopped greens such as kale or chard

1 pound chicken breast

2 cups chicken broth

1 cup coconut milk

2 cups riced cauliflower

To serve: hot sauce shredded coconut, lime wedges

Sea salt and fresh ground pepper to taste

## METHOD

### STEP 1

Heat the oil in a large pot or Dutch oven to medium high heat. Add the onion, garlic, and ginger, and cook until softened. Stir in the curry powder and greens and cook until greens are softened. Add the curry powder, chicken breast, and broth. Bring to a boil and reduce to a simmer.

### STEP 2

Simmer until chicken is cooked through. Remove breasts from pot and shred with two forks. Return to the pot and add the coconut milk and cauliflower. Simmer for 5 minutes. Serve immediately.

## NUTRITION VALUE

435 Kcal, 20g fat, 3.3g fiber, 29.5g protein, 10.1g carbs.

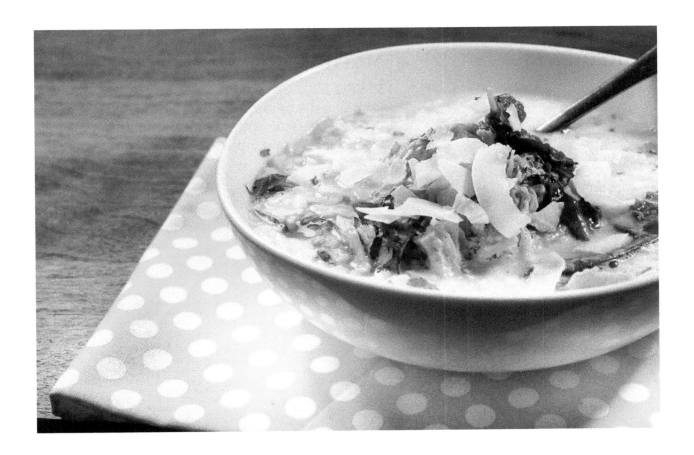

# LEMON CAPER TUNA WRAPS

se easy lettuce wraps require pretty much that same amount of effort as opening a can of tuna, but they are loaded with flavor, thanks in part to caper berries, tiny round berries that are pickled to be salty and briny. Perfect with tuna.

MAKES 1 SERVING/ TOTAL TIME 10 MINUTE

## INGREDIENTS

1 5 oz can of tuna drained

1 tablespoons olive oil

Juice and zest of 1 lemon

1 tablespoon capers

1 tablespoon fresh chopped parsley

1 clove garlic minced

2 firm crisp lettuce leaves left intact

1/4 cup diced tomatoes

Sea salt and fresh ground pepper to taste

## METHOD

### STEP 1
Combine the tuna, oil, lemon , capers, parsley and garlic in a bowl. Season with salt and pepper. Spoon into the lettuce leaves and top with the tomatoes before serving.

## NUTRITION VALUE

467 Kcal, 20g fat,
1g fiber, 48.1g protein, 3.4g carbs.

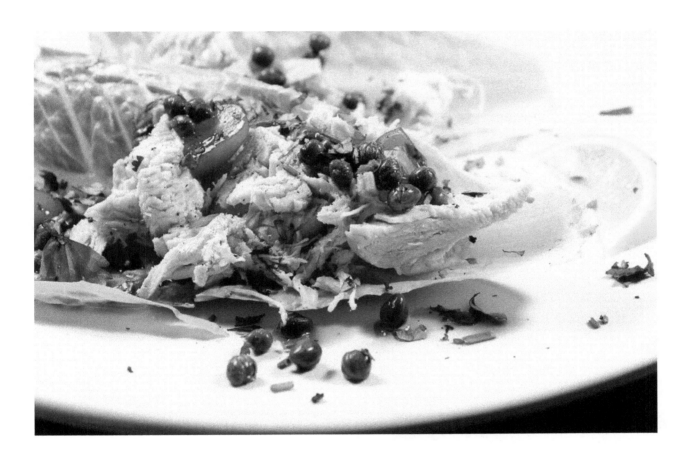

# CAULIFLOWER RICE STEAK BOWL

A quick and easy bowl filled with tender beef, caramelized Brussels sprouts and cauliflower rice makes the perfect healthy lunch option.

MAKES 2 SERVING/ TOTAL TIME 20 MINUTE

## INGREDIENTS

3 tablespoons olive oil

10 ounces sirloin steak cubed

1 pound Brussels sprouts cored and halved

2 cups riced cauliflower

Juice of 1 lemon

1/4 cup sliced almonds

Sea salt and fresh ground pepper to taste

## METHOD

### STEP 1

Heat the oil in a heavy skillet over medium heat. Add the steak and cook until well browned. Remove from pan, leaving as much of the fat behind as possible. Add the Brussels sprouts cut side down and sear until well browned.

### STEP 2

Flip and continue cooking for another minute or two. Add the cauliflower and cook until softened. Add the lemon juice, almonds, and steak and cook until heated through. Serve immediately.

**NUTRITION VALUE**

625 Kcal, 20 fat, 11g fiber, 54.2g protein, 14 carbs.

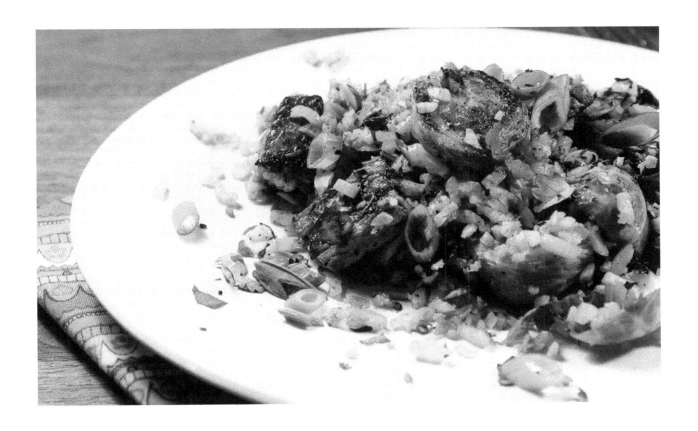

# JUICY ITALIAN CHICKEN BREAST

Take the guesswork out of chicken breasts with this easy, fast recipe. Serve these with your favorite veggies or slice and add to a big green salad for a healthy meal in a flash.

MAKES 4 SERVING/ TOTAL TIME 10 MINUTE

## INGREDIENTS

4 6-ounce chicken breasts

1 teaspoon Italian seasoning

2 tablespoons olive oil

1 cup chicken broth or water

Juice of 1 lemon

Sea salt and fresh ground pepper to taste

## METHOD

### STEP 1

Season your chicken with the Italian seasoning and salt and pepper. Using the sauté setting on your Instant Pot, add the oil and the chicken breasts, and cook for about 2 minutes per side. Remove from the pot and add the broth or water to the bottom.

### STEP 2

Set the steamer rack in the pot and add the chicken to the rack. Drizzle with the lemon juice.

Close your pot and set your timer to 5 minutes at high pressure.

Remove the chicken and allow to rest for a few minutes before serving.

**NUTRITION  VALUE**

467 Kcal, 20g fat,
1g fiber, 48.1g protein, 3.4g carbs.

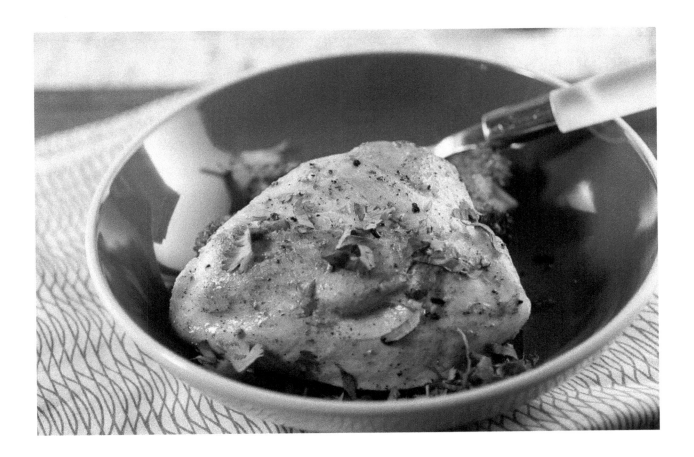

# LEMON CHICKEN BRUSSELS SPROUT SALAD

When paired with chicken, bacon, and a tangy lemon dressing, it turns lunch time into something you'll look forward to.

MAKES 4 SERVING/ TOTAL TIME 20 MINUTE

## INGREDIENTS

4 slices bacon chopped

1 pound chicken breasts

1 pound Brussels sprouts cored and finely shredded

1/2 cup olive oil

Juice and zest of 1 lemon

1 teaspoon Dijon mustard

1 clove garlic minced

Sea salt and fresh ground pepper to taste

## METHOD

### STEP 1

Heat a skillet to medium heat and cook the bacon pieces until crisp. Remove with a slotted spoon, leaving the fat behind. Add the chicken and cook until browned and cooked through. Remove the chicken from the pan and let cool, then shred with two forks.

### STEP 2

Put the sprouts in a bowl with the bacon. Add the chicken. Put the remaining ingredients in a jar and shake until well combined. Toss with the salad and serve.

**NUTRITION VALUE**

544 Kcal, 20g fat,
0.8g fiber, 40.6g protein, 2.3g carbs.

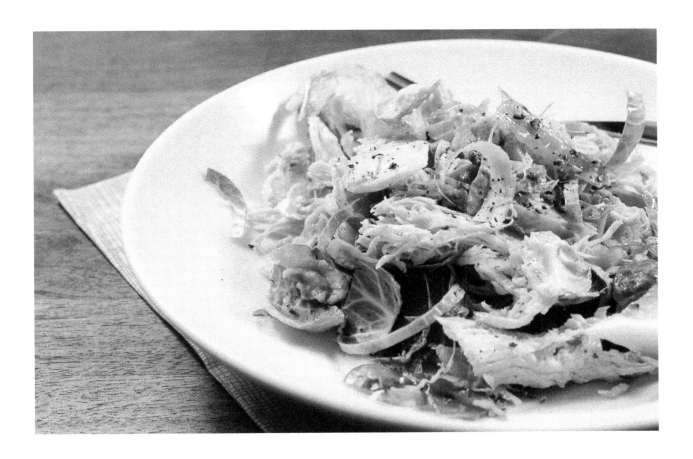

# Dinner

# PALEO CHICKEN COLOMBO RECIPE

Roasted bone-in chicken thighs may be served up **Greek-style with black olives** and cherry tomatoes.

MAKES 4 SERVING/ TOTAL TIME 60 MINUTE

## INGREDIENTS

8 chicken thighs, skinless with bone-in

3 sweet potatoes, peeled and cubed

1 zucchini, cubed

2 green onions, sliced

3 cloves garlic, minced

1 tbsp. fresh ginger, minced

2 cups full-fat coconut milk

2 tbsp. fresh lime juice

1/2 tsp. ground coriander

1/2 tsp. ground mustard

1/2 tsp. ground cumin

1/2 tsp. ground aniseed

1/2 tsp. ground ginger

2 tbsp. coconut oil

## METHOD

### STEP 1

In a bowl combine the coriander, mustard, cumin, aniseed, and ginger. Season the chicken to taste with sea salt and freshly ground black pepper.

Melt some coconut oil in a Dutch oven over medium-high heat, brown the chicken pieces on both sides, about 4 minutes, then set aside.

In the same pot, add the onion and garlic; cook 2 to 3 minutes.

### STEP 2

Add all the remaining vegetables and cook another 2 to 3 minutes. Pour in the coconut milk, lime juice, and the coriander mixture, then give everything a good stir.

Return the chicken to the pot and season everything to taste.

Cover and simmer 40 to 45 minutes, stirring occasionally, or until chicken is fully cooked.

**NUTRITION  VALUE**

806 Kcal, 20g fat,
13.6g fiber, 59g protein, 14g carbs.

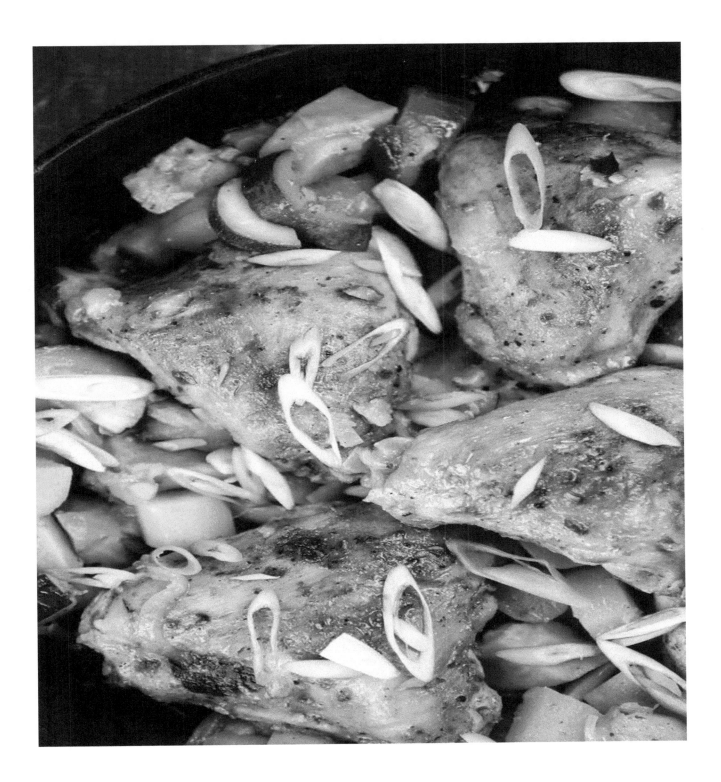

# PUMPKIN SPICED CHICKEN THIGHS

Pumpkin spice is good for more than just lattes and pies. It spices up chicken thighs nicely, as seen here. Serve with braised greens and mashed cauliflower for a delicious and healthy

MAKES 4 SERVING/ TOTAL TIME 40 MINUTE

## INGREDIENTS

2 pounds chicken thighs

1 tablespoon pumpkin pie spice

3 tablespoons olive oil

Sea salt and fresh ground pepper to taste

## METHOD

### STEP 1

Preheat oven to 350 degrees F.

Heat a heavy, deep, ovenproof skillet over medium high heat. Season the chicken with the pumpkin pie spice, and liberally sprinkle with salt and pepper. Add the chicken to the pan and cook until well browned.

### STEP 2

Flip and transfer to oven and continue cooking until chicken has reached an internal temperature of 165 degrees.

Let rest for 5 minutes and serve.

| NUTRITION VALUE | 413 Kcal, 19g fat, 43g protein, 2g carbs. |
|---|---|

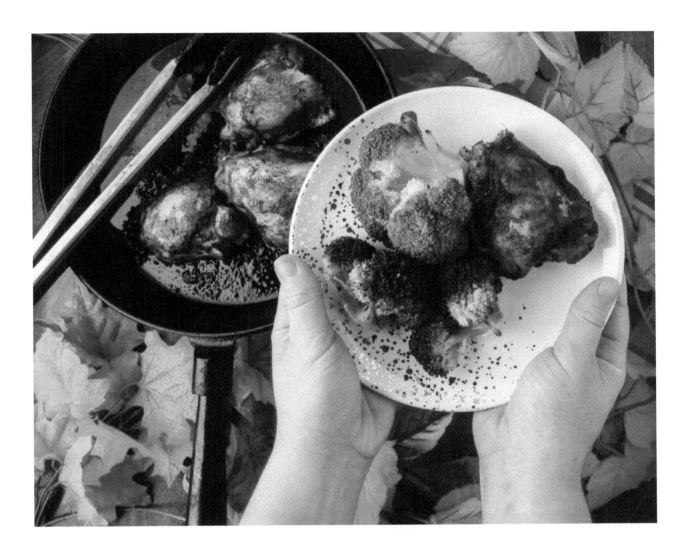

# LEMON HERB GRILLED CHICKEN

A quick lemon herb sauce turns chicken breasts into a masterpiece. Delicious for an outdoor meal or sliced on top of a salad.

MAKES 4 SERVING/ TOTAL TIME  4 HOU R 30 MINUTE

## INGREDIENTS

1/4 cup olive oil

1 bunch parsley

5 green onions

4 basil leaves

2 cloves garlic

1 teaspoon salt

Juice and zest of 1 lemon

4 chicken breasts

## METHOD

### STEP 1

Put everything but the chicken in a blender and blend until smooth. Marinate the chicken for 2-4 hours.

### STEP 2

When ready to grill, preheat gas or charcoal grill to medium high heat. Grill chicken until internal temperature reaches 165 degrees.
Let chicken rest for 5 minutes before serving.

**NUTRITION  VALUE**

278 Kcal, 15g fat,
2g fiber, 30g protein, 2g carbs.

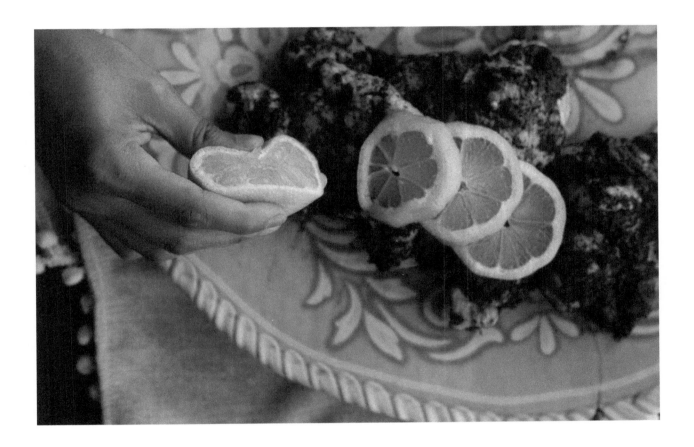

# GRILLED FLANK STEAK WITH CHIMICHURRI

An herby marinade turns flank steak into an amazing meal, perfect for sitting on the patio on a nice night. Serve this with your favorite veggies for a nutritious meal.

MAKES 4 SERVING/ TOTAL TIME 2 HOUR

## INGREDIENTS

1 bunch parsley

1 bunch cilantro

3 cloves garlic

1 teaspoon crushed red pepper flakes

1 teaspoon oregano

Juice and zest of 1 lemon

1 cup olive oil

1 teaspoon sea salt

1/2 teaspoon black pepper

2 pounds flank steak

## METHOD

### STEP 1

Put the parsley, cilantro, garlic, pepper flakes, oregano, lemon, salt, and pepper in a blender and blend until smooth. Put the steak in a freezer bag or casserole dish. Pour half the chimichurri over the steak and marinate for at least 30 minutes.

### STEP 2

When ready to cook, preheat grill to medium high heat. Grill the steak until done to your liking.

Let rest for 5-10 minutes, and then slice the steak against the grain.

Serve the steak topped with the reserved chimichurri.

### NUTRITION VALUE

940Kcal, 20g fat, 9g fiber, 47g protein, 4g carbs.

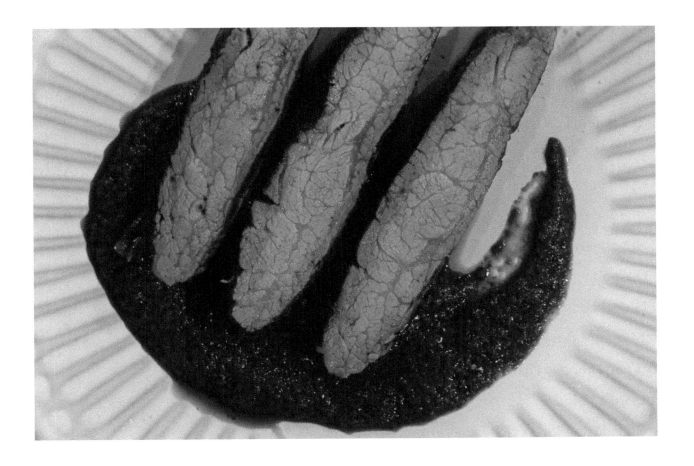

# THAI CHICKEN CURRY

Spicy and fragrant, this easy curried is the perfect alternative to sodium and carb filled takeout. You can sub shrimp for the chicken if you'd like for a change of pace.

MAKES 4 SERVING/ TOTAL TIME 30 MINUTE

## INGREDIENTS

2 tablespoons coconut oil

1 1/2 pounds chicken breast sliced

1 onion diced

1 chili pepper minced

1 carrot diced

2 cloves garlic minced

1 teaspoon grated fresh ginger

2 tablespoons Thai red curry paste

1 14- ounce can coconut milk

1/4 cup chopped cilantro

Juice of 1 lime

Steamed cauliflower rice for serving

Sea salt and fresh ground pepper to taste

## METHOD
### STEP 1

Heat the oil in a heavy pot over medium high heat and add the chicken. Cook until browned and add the onion, pepper, and carrot. Continue cooking until softened, and add the garlic and ginger. Cook for another minute, stir in the curry paste, and coconut milk.

### STEP 2

Bring to a simmer, and simmer for 5 minutes.

Stir in the cilantro and lime juice, and serve over the cauliflower rice.

## NUTRITION  VALUE

400 Kcal, 19g fat, 6g fiber, 38g protein, 14.9g carbs.

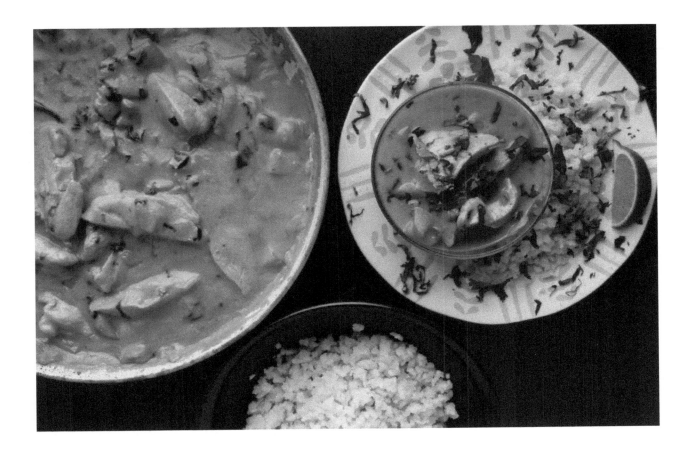

# BRAISED SHORT RIBS WITH GARLIC ROSEMARY MASHED CAULIFLOWER

Short ribs are an upscale version of pot roast, and perfect for a romantic celebration or when you just want a fancy dinner.

MAKES 2 SERVING/ TOTAL TIME 3 HOUR

## INGREDIENTS

3 slices bacon diced

2 tablespoons olive oil

4 beef short ribs

1 small onion diced

1 shallot minced

1 carrot diced

2 cups chicken or beef broth

1 sprig thyme

1 sprig parsley

1 sprig rosemary

2 cloves garlic smashed

4 cups cauliflower florets

2 cloves garlic smashed

1/4 cup buttermilk or coconut milk

2 tablespoons butter

## METHOD

### STEP 1

Preheat oven to 350 degrees F. In a heavy pot or Dutch oven, cook the bacon until crisp. Remove from pan with a slotted spoon.  Add the olive oil and cook the onion, shallots, and carrot until softened, scraping the browned bits from the bottom. Add the short ribs back to the pot, along with the broth. Add additional water if necessary to make sure short ribs are about 3/4 covered. Add the herbs and garlic cloves and cover. Put in the oven and cook for about 2 hours. Turn the heat down and cook for another 45 minutes, or until ribs are falling apart with a fork.

### STEP 2

First, steam the florets and garlic cloves until very soft, either in a vegetable steamer basket or the microwave. Put the cauliflower and garlic in a food processor with the milk and half the butter. Puree until smooth and creamy and stir in the remaining butter and rosemary before serving. Serve .

**NUTRITION  VALUE**

713 Kcal, 21g fat,
4g fiber, 48g protein, 14.9g carbs.

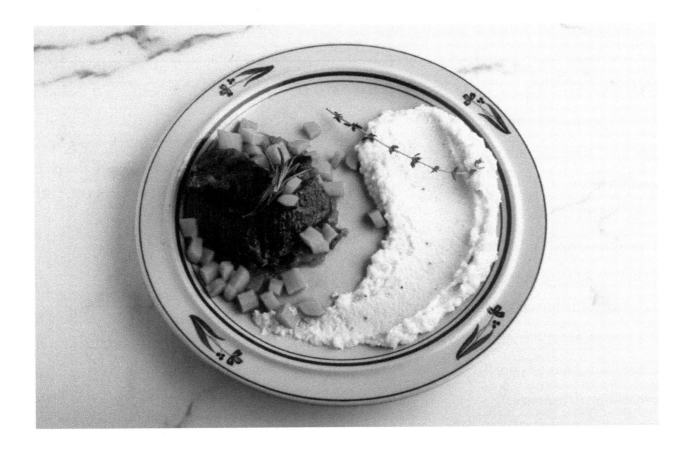

# LAMB AND ROOT VEGETABLE STEW

Hearty and full of chunky vegetables, this stew is rich with flavor, full of good fat and antioxidants, and most importantly delicious. Perfect for a cold winter night when you want something comforting, but without refined carbs.

MAKES 2  SERVING/ TOTAL TIME  1 HOUR 10 MINUTE

## INGREDIENTS

2 tablespoons olive oil

2 pounds lamb shoulder cubed

1 onion diced

2 carrots diced

2 turnips peeled and cubed

2 parsnips peeled and cubed

3 cloves garlic minced

1 teaspoon ground cumin

1 teaspoon smoked paprika

1 teaspoon dried parsley

2 tablespoons tomato paste

6 cups chicken or beef broth

2 bay leaves

1 tablespoon apple cider vinegar

Sea salt and fresh ground pepper to taste

## METHOD

### STEP 1

Heat the olive oil in a heavy pot or Dutch oven. Season the lamb with salt and pepper and add it to the pot. Cook until well browned and remove from pot. Set aside.

### STEP 2

Add the veggies to the pot and cook until softened. Stir in the garlic and seasonings and continue cooking for another minute. Add the tomato paste, stir, and add the lamb back to the pot.

Add the broth and bay leaves, and bring to a boil. Reduce to a simmer and simmer on medium low heat for an hour, or until lamb is tender. Add the apple cider vinegar and remove the bay leaves.

Serve immediately.

| NUTRITION  VALUE | 740 Kcal, 20g fat, 8g fiber, 50g protein, 14g carbs. |
|---|---|

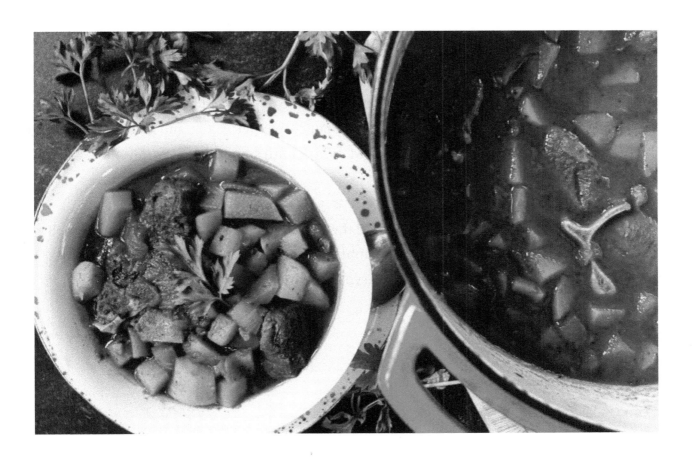

# CHOPPED CHICKEN SALAD WITH SESAME ALMOND DRESSING

A creamy almond dressing takes a simple salad to a new level. This salad will show you just how amazing a salad can be.

MAKES 2 SERVING/ TOTAL TIME 20 MINUTE

## INGREDIENTS

1/2 cup toasted sesame oil

1/4 cup almond butter

1 teaspoon ginger

1 clove garlic grated

Juice and zest of 1 orange

1/2 teaspoon crushed red pepper flakes

1 teaspoon Paleo approved fish sauce

4 cups shredded cabbage

1/2 cup shredded carrots

4 green onions sliced

1 orange segmented

2 cups cooked and diced chicken breast

1/2 cup sliced almonds

## METHOD

### STEP 1

Put the sesame oil, almond butter, ginger, garlic, orange zest and juice, pepper flakes, and fish sauce in a large bowl. Whisk until smooth and creamy.

### STEP 2

Add the remaining ingredients and toss until well combined.

Serve immediately.

| NUTRITION  VALUE | 1213 Kcal, 20g fat, 13g fiber, 84g protein, 14.9g carbs. |
|---|---|

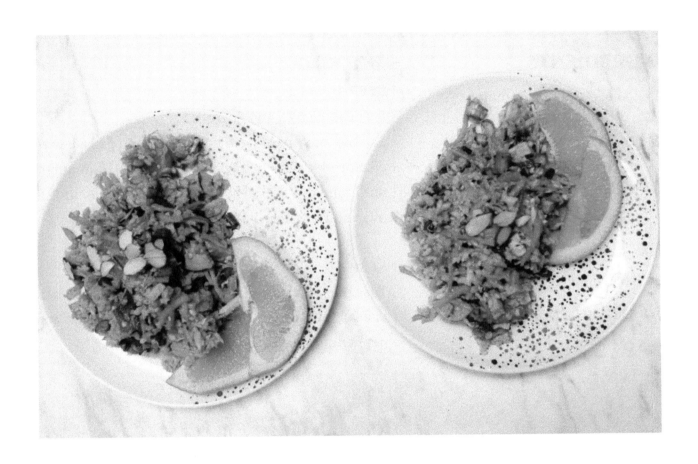

# ROASTED TOMATOES TUNA AND ZOODLES

Recipe that everyone love.

MAKES 2 SERVING/ TOTAL TIME 20 MINUTE

## INGREDIENTS

1 cup halved cherry tomatoes

1 tablespoon olive oil

1/2 teaspoon dried thyme

2 zucchini cut into noodles

2 cans tuna drained and flaked

Juice of 1 lemon

2 tablespoons fresh chopped basil

Sea salt and fresh ground pepper to taste

## METHOD

**STEP 1**

Preheat oven to 400 degrees F.

Lay the tomatoes on a baking sheet and drizzle with the oil. Sprinkle with thyme and roast for 8-10 minutes, until tomatoes are shriveled and sizzling. Remove from oven and let cool.

**STEP 2**

Toss the noodles, tuna, lemon juice, basil, and tomatoes in a large bowl until combined. Season with salt and pepper and serve.

**NUTRITION VALUE**

163 Kcal, 10g fat,
4g fiber, 20g protein, 12g carbs.

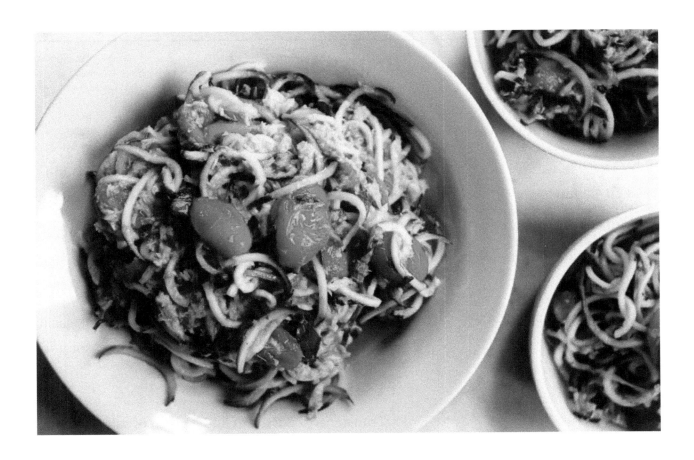

# PESTO CHICKEN STUFFED CHICKEN BREASTS

Our version is as simple as you can get – basil leaves, walnuts, garlic, and olive oil

MAKES 2 SERVING/ TOTAL TIME 60 MINUTE

## INGREDIENTS

2 medium sweet potatoes

1/2 cup packed basil leaves

1 clove garlic

1/4 cup walnuts

1/4 cup olive oil

2 cups cooked and shredded chicken

sea salt to taste

fresh ground pepper to taste

## METHOD

### STEP 1

Preheat oven to 400 degrees F.

Put the potatoes on a sheet pan and bake for 30 minutes. Remove from oven, prick with a fork and continue baking another 30 minutes or so, until a knife slides into the potatoes with no resistance. Remove and let cool slightly.

### STEP 2

While potatoes are baking, combine the basil, garlic, walnuts, and oil in a blender or food processor and pulse until blended.

Transfer to a bowl and add a pinch of salt and pepper, and add the chicken. Mix well.

Split the potatoes open and stuff with the chicken mixture.

Serve immediately.

## NUTRITION VALUE

163 Kcal, 10g fat,
4g fiber, 20g protein, 12g carbs.

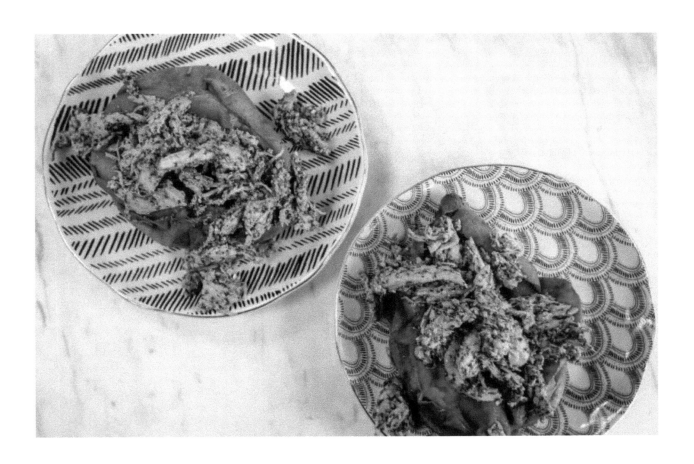

# ITALIAN BEEF AND BROCCOLI

With garlic, basil, Italian seasoning, and a squeeze of lemon, there is no lack of flavor in this dish. It will surely make it into your dinner rotation!

MAKES 2 SERVING/ TOTAL TIME 20 MINUTE

## INGREDIENTS

2 tablespoons olive oil

1 clove garlic minced

2 basil leaves slivered

12 ounces sliced beef

2 cups broccoli florets

1 teaspoon Italian seasoning

1 tablespoon lemon juice

Grated Parmesan optional, for serving

Sea salt and fresh ground pepper to taste

## METHOD

**STEP 1**

Heat the oil in a heavy skillet. Add the garlic and basil and cook for about a minute. Add the beef, cook until browned, and add the broccoli. Continue cooking until softened.

**STEP 2**

Add the Italian seasoning and lemon juice, and remove from heat.

Sprinkle with the Parmesan if using.

**NUTRITION  VALUE**

353 Kcal, 15g fat,
8g fiber, 35g protein, 15g carbs.

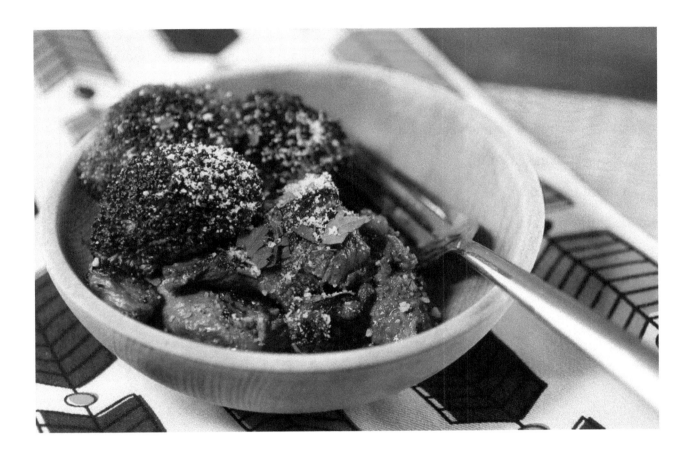

# ITALIAN BEEF SOUP

This flavorful soup comes together in a flash. It's healthy, comforting, and perfect for a cold winter day when you want dinner fast.

MAKES 6 SERVING/ TOTAL TIME 1 5MINUTE

## INGREDIENTS

1.5 pounds grass-fed ground beef

1 onion sliced

2 cloves garlic chopped

1 head kale or bunch spinach chopped

1 teaspoon Italian seasoning

1 can diced tomatoes

4 cups chicken broth

2 cups water

2 carrots sliced

Juice of 1 lemon

Sea salt and fresh ground pepper to taste

## METHOD

### STEP 1

Using your sauté setting, cook the beef until no longer pink in the center. Remove the beef and add the onions and garlic. Cook for 2 minutes.

### STEP 2

Add the remaining ingredients to the pot, and close the lid. Set timer to 5 minutes at high pressure and cook. Serve immediately.

## NUTRITION VALUE

553 Kcal, 9g fat,
7g fiber, 56g protein, 14g carbs.

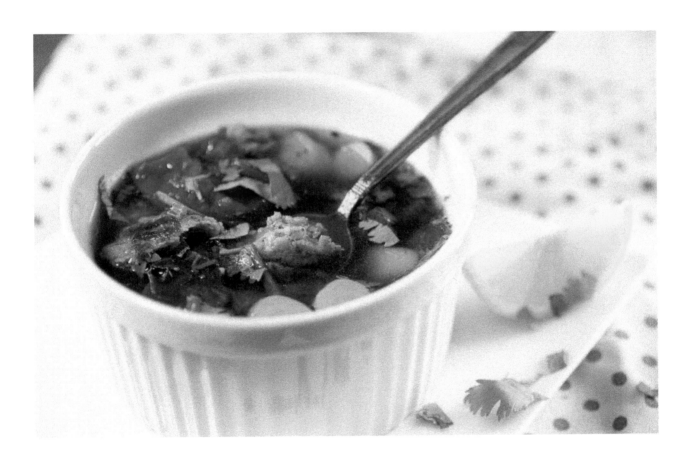

# Desserts

# BERRY CHIA SMOOTHIE BOWL

Frozen berries are sweet and juicy, and blend up into a brightly colored, beautiful bowl of goodness. Topped with your favorite nuts and seeds, you'll want to make this every day.

MAKES 2 SERVING/ TOTAL TIME 10 MINUTE

## INGREDIENTS

2 cups frozen mixed berries

1 banana chopped

2 tablespoons chia seeds

3 tablespoons almond milk

Toppings: coconut flakes chia seeds, fresh berries, chopped nuts

## METHOD

### STEP 1

Put the berries, banana and chia seeds in a blender and begin blending on low. Slowly add the almond milk and increase blending speed until mixture is thick and smooth.

Transfer to bowls and top with desired toppings. Serve immediately.

**NUTRITION  VALUE**

200 Kcal, 10g fat,
10g fiber, 20g protein, 15g carbs.

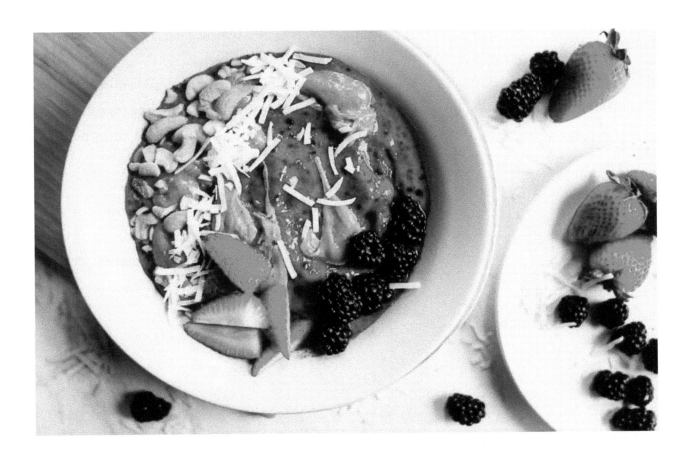

# CINNAMON HONEY GRANOLA

Recipe that Everyone love.

MAKES 4 SERVING/ TOTAL TIME 1 HOUR

## INGREDIENTS

1 cup almonds

1 cup pecans

.5 cup walnuts

.25 cup sunflower seeds

2 tbsp sesame seeds

1 tsp cinnamon

1 tsp sea salt

.25 cup honey

.25 cup coconut oil

1 tsp vanilla extract

.25 cup raisins or cranberries

## METHOD

**STEP 1**

Preheat oven to 300 degrees F. Line a large baking sheet with parchment paper.

 Put the nuts, seeds, cinnamon, and salt in a large bowl. In a small saucepan, combine the honey, coconut oil, and vanilla. Heat on low until melted and smooth. Pour over the nuts and stir to coat.

**STEP 2**

Transfer mixture to baking sheet and bake for 40 minutes, stirring halfway through.

Remove from oven and let cool completely. Break into small pieces or pulse in a food processor for a finer texture.

Store leftovers in an airtight container.

**NUTRITION  VALUE**

335 Kcal, 14g fat,
8g fiber, 32g protein, 15g carbs.

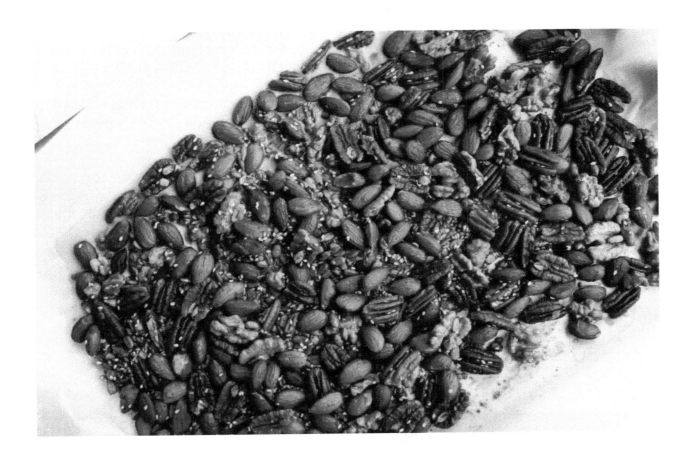

# DARK CHOCOLATE ALMOND BLONDIES

Decadent, dark, and delicious – all of these adjectives perfectly describe these dark chocolate almond blondies.

MAKES 16 SERVING/ TOTAL TIME 45 MINUTE

## INGREDIENTS

1/2 cup almond butter

1/4 cup melted coconut oil

3/4 cup coconut sugar

1 egg

1 tbsp vanilla extract

1 cup almond flour

1 tsp baking soda

1/2 tsp kosher salt

1/2 cup chopped dark chocolate

## METHOD

**STEP 1**
Preheat oven to 350 degrees F.
Put the almond butter, coconut oil, coconut sugar, egg, and vanilla in a large bowl. Whisk until smooth and well combined.
In a separate bowl, combine the almond flour, baking soda, salt, and chocolate. Add this to the wet ingredients and mix well.

**STEP 2**
Spray a square baking dish with cooking spray and spread the batter evenly in it. Bake for 20-25 minutes until a toothpick inserted in the center comes out clean.
Allow to cool completely and cut into 16 squares.

**NUTRITION  VALUE**

335 Kcal, 14g fat,
8g fiber, 32g protein, 15g carbs.

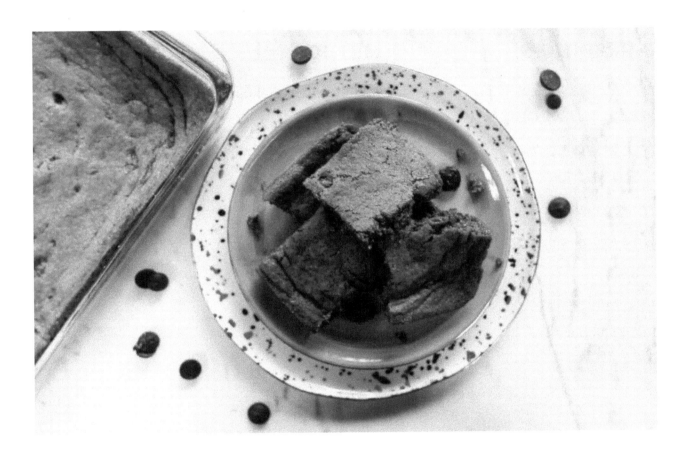

# BLUEBERRY MUFFINS

These paleo-friendly blueberry muffins will do the trick. They come together easily with almond flour, coconut sugar, coconut oil, and a whole lotta love.

MAKES 12 SERVING/ TOTAL TIME 40 MINUTE

## INGREDIENTS

2.5 cup almond flour

1/2 cup coconut sugar

2 tsp baking powder

1/2 tsp sea salt

1/3 cup melted coconut oil

1/3 cup non-dairy milk

3 eggs

1 tsp vanilla extract

1 cup blueberries

## METHOD
**STEP 1**
Preheat oven to 350 degrees F. Line a muffin pan with paper liners.
Combine the almond flour, coconut sugar, baking powder, and salt in a bowl and mix well.

**STEP 2**
Add the oil, milk, eggs, and vanilla and stir to combine. Fold in the blueberries.
Fill the muffin tin until about 2/3 full.
Bake for 20-23 minutes, until tops are golden brown and a toothpick inserted comes out clean. Let cool before serving.

**NUTRITION  VALUE**

335 Kcal, 14g fat,
8g fiber, 32g protein, 15g carbs.

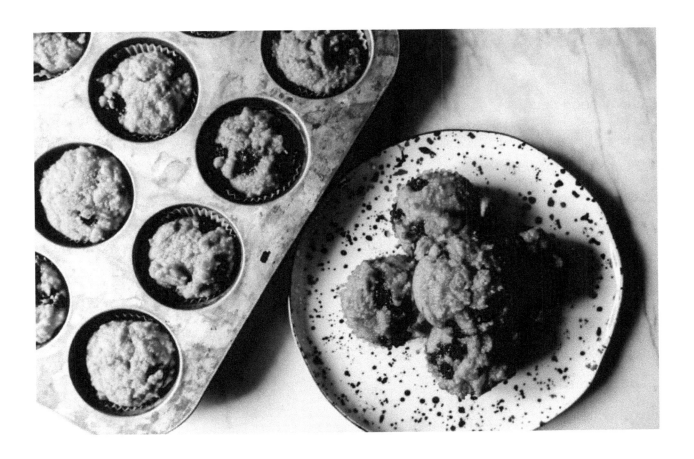

# SLOW COOKER CHOCOLATE STRAWBERRY CAKE

This decadent cake takes a few hours, but requires no hands-on time, and is elegant and delicious. It's proof your slow cooker is for more than just stews and roasts.

**MAKES 8 SERVING/ TOTAL TIME 3 HOUR**

## INGREDIENTS

Cake:

1 cup almond flour

1/2 cup honey

1/2 cup cocoa powder

1 teaspoon baking powder

1/2 teaspoon sea salt

3 eggs

6 tablespoons coconut oil

2/3 cup coconut milk

1 teaspoon vanilla

1 cup diced strawberries

Frosting:

1/2 cup finely chopped dark chocolate

1/2 cup coconut milk

## METHOD

### STEP 1

Whisk all of the ingredients for the cake together in your slow cooker pot. Cover and cook on low for 2-3 hours, until cake is done. Cool completely.

### STEP 2

To make the frosting, combine the chocolate and coconut milk in a saucepan and heat over low heat until chocolate is melted. Spread over cooled cake.

**NUTRITION  VALUE**

323 Kcal, 10g fat,
8g fiber, 36g protein, 15g carbs.

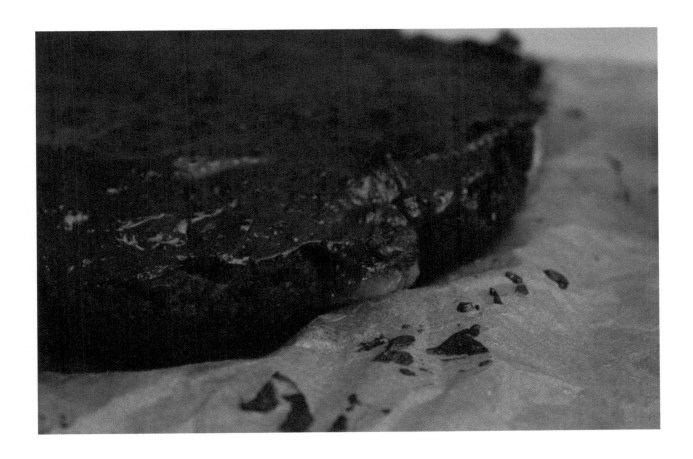

# BLUEBERRY PANCAKE SCONES

This recipe utilizes almond and coconut flour as well as maple syrup and sugar.

MAKES 6 SERVING/ TOTAL TIME 30 MINUTE

## INGREDIENTS

2 cups almond flour

3 tablespoons coconut flour

1/4 cup maple syrup

1 egg

1/4 cup coconut or almond milk

3 tablespoons coconut oil

1/2 teaspoon baking soda

1/4 teaspoon sea salt

1 cup blueberries

1 tablespoon maple sugar

## METHOD

**STEP 1**

Preheat oven to 350 degrees F.

Combine the flours, maple syrup, egg, oil, baking soda, and salt in a mixing bowl. Stir until a dough forms, and fold in the blueberries.

**STEP 2**

Transfer the mixture to a clean surface, and form into a 3-inch-thick circle. Cut into wedges and transfer to a parchment lined baking sheet.

Sprinkle with the maple sugar and bake until gold brown, 15-18 minutes.

**NUTRITION  VALUE**

503 Kcal, 11g fat,
7g fiber, 36g protein, 15g carbs.

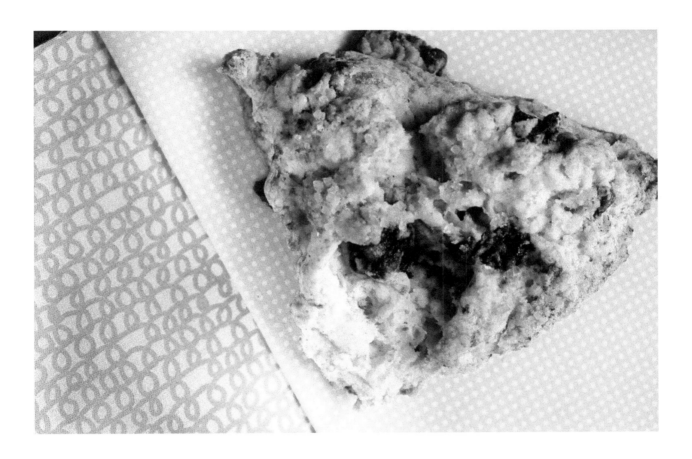

# Snacks

# TUNA CUCUMBER BITES

These easy no-cook appetizers come together fast, and they taste delicious. The tuna salad can be made ahead of time and everything can be put together right before you need it.

MAKES 1 SERVING/ TOTAL TIME 20 MINUTE

## INGREDIENTS

2 (5 oz) cans high-quality tuna drained

1/2 cup finely minced onion

2 cloves garlic minced

2 tablespoons fresh chopped dill

1 tablespoon lemon juice

2 seedless cucumbers thinly sliced

Sea salt and fresh ground pepper to taste

## METHOD
### STEP 1
Combine the tuna, onion, garlic, dill, and lemon juice in a bowl and mix well.

Lay the cucumber slices on a sheet tray or serving platter and top with the tuna mixture. Serve at room temperature.

**NUTRITION  VALUE**

625 Kcal, 20 fat, 11g fiber, 54.2g protein, 14 carbs.

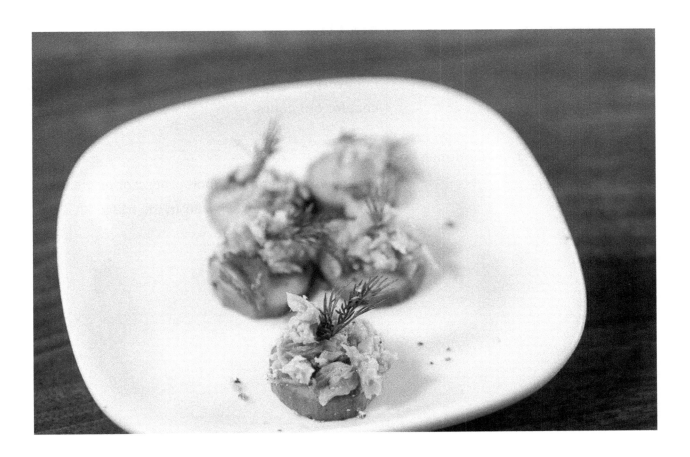

# SPICED APPLE PEAR SAUCE

Pears give the usual applesauce a new dimension of flavor. Better than anything you'll buy in the store, this is perfect for breakfast, as a side, or used in baked goods.

MAKES 1 SERVING/ TOTAL TIME 6 HOUR

## INGREDIENTS

3 large apples peeled and cored

3 large pears peeled and cored

2 cinnamon sticks

1/8 teaspoon fresh grated nutmeg

1 teaspoon vanilla

Pinch of salt

## METHOD

### STEP 1

Put everything in your slow cooker and cook over low heat for 6-8 hours.

### STEP 2

Mash well or blend in a food processor or blender. Cool completely, and store in a jar in the fridge

## NUTRITION VALUE

358 Kcal, 20g fat,
4.5g fiber, 26.1g protein, 11.6g carbs.

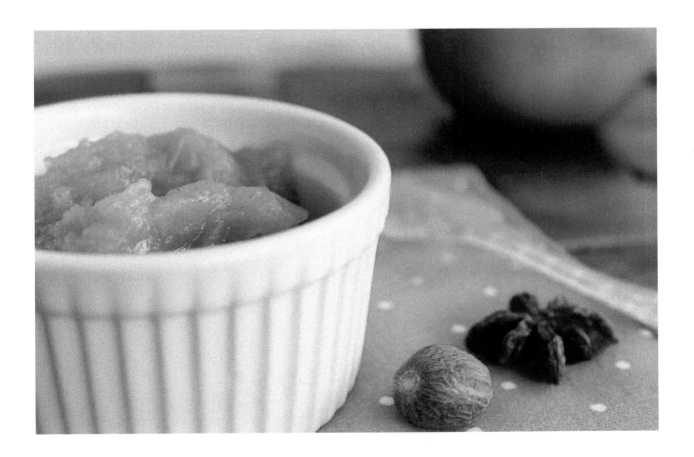

# MARINATED RAW FETA

This easy appetizer is rich and flavorful and couldn't be easier to make. Serve with olives, sundried tomatoes, and high-quality cured meat for amazing appetizers your guests will love.

MAKES 1 SERVING/ TOTAL TIME 30 MINUTE

## INGREDIENTS

8 ounces raw feta cheese sliced into 1/2" slabs

1 cup extra-virgin olive oil

2 cloves garlic smashed

2 sprigs fresh mint

2 sprigs fresh oregano

1 lemon juiced

1 teaspoon whole peppercorns

1 teaspoon crushed red pepper flakes optional

## METHOD

### STEP 1

Lay the cheese in a shallow container. Add the remaining ingredients, making sure the cheese is covered by the oil.

Cover and refrigerate for several hours, but up to 3 days. Serve at room temperature.

**NUTRITION  VALUE**

498 Kcal, 20g fat,
3.9g fiber, 21.7g protein, 15g carbs.

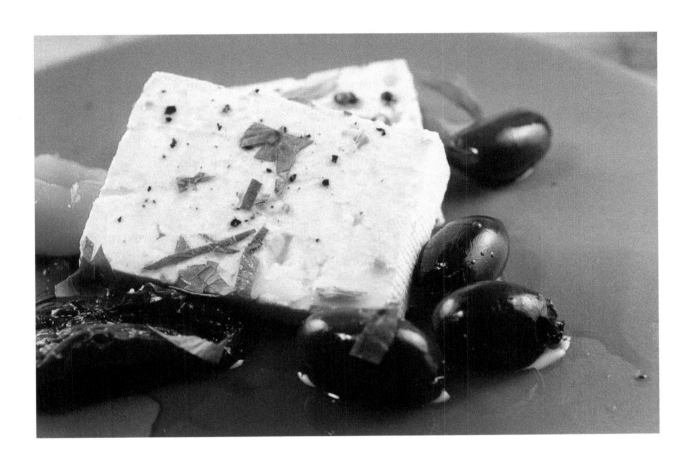

# BONE BROTH

Homemade bone broth is loaded with nutrients, but is not a quick process. With your Instant Pot, that changes. This easy recipe is versatile, nutritious, and perfect for soups, stews, or even just drinking out of a mug on a cold day.

MAKES 8 SERVING/ TOTAL TIME 2 HOUR

## INGREDIENTS

3 pounds bones of your choice chicken, beef, or pork, or mix

1 onion halved

4 stalks celery

2 carrots peeled and cut into chunks

Fresh herbs: parsley rosemary, or thyme

lemon juiced

Water

1 tablespoon kosher salt

## METHOD

### STEP 1

Put the bones in your instant pot with your veggies, herbs, and lemon juice.

Cover with about 8 cups of water, but don't fill your pot more than about 2/3 full. Add salt.

### STEP 2

Lock the lid and cook at high pressure for about 2 hours. Use the natural release to release the pressure.

Allow to cool and strain the broth. Store in sealed containers in the fridge, or freeze for longer storage.

## NUTRITION  VALUE

464 Kcal, 20g fat, 20.8g fiber, 43g protein, 8g carbs.

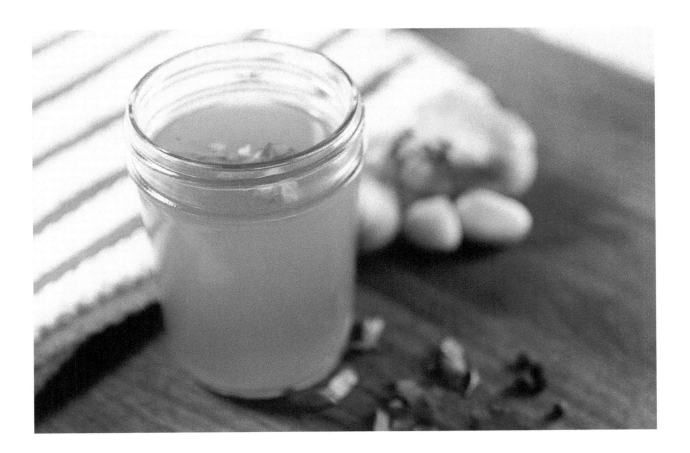

# CURRIED ROASTED CAULIFLOWER

Spicy and flavorful, this easy side dish adds exotic flair to anything you serve it with.

MAKES 4 SERVING/ TOTAL TIME 30 MINUTE

## INGREDIENTS

1 head cauliflower cut into florets

1/2 cup fresh or frozen peas

1 tablespoon curry powder

2 tablespoons coconut oil

Sea salt and fresh ground pepper to taste

## METHOD

**STEP 1**

Preheat oven to 400 degrees F.

Toss the cauliflower and peas with the curry and coconut oil. Lay on a baking sheet and roast for 30 minutes, or until tender.

Serve immediately.

**NUTRITION VALUE**

197 Kcal, 13g fat, 5.8g fiber, 10g protein, 14.8g carbs.

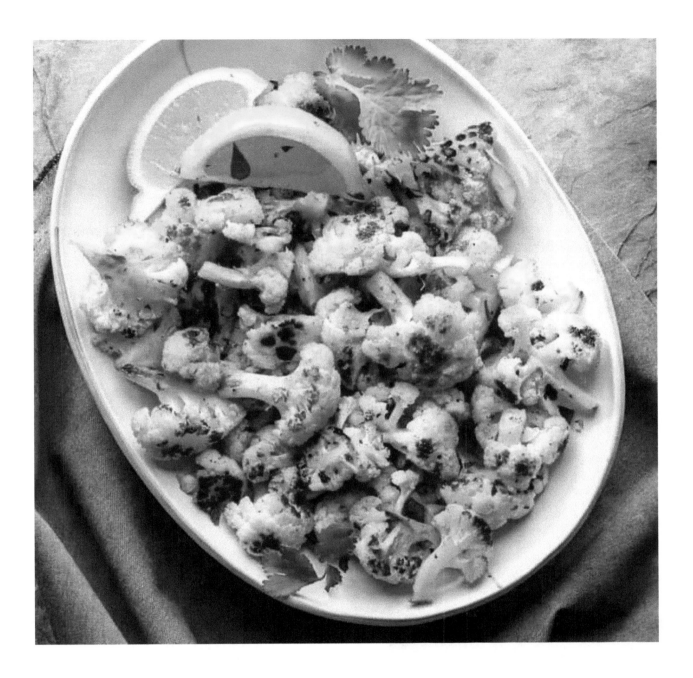

# PALEO SLIDERS

You don't need a bun to have a delicious slider. If you're serving these at a party, stick toothpicks in them so guests can easily pick up and go.

MAKES 1 SERVING/ TOTAL TIME 30 MINUTE

## INGREDIENTS

1-pound grass-fed ground beef

1/2-pound ground veal

1 egg

1/4 cup almond flour

2 cloves garlic minced

1/4 cup finely minced onion

1 teaspoon Italian seasoning

## METHOD

**STEP 1**

Mix all of the ingredients in a bowl using your hands, being careful not to over mix.

**STEP 2**

Form into 2-inch patties, and cook in a skillet until cooked through. Serve with your favorite Paleo condiments like mayo or mustard.

**NUTRITION  VALUE**

197 Kcal, 13g fat,
5.8g fiber, 10g protein, 14.8g carbs.

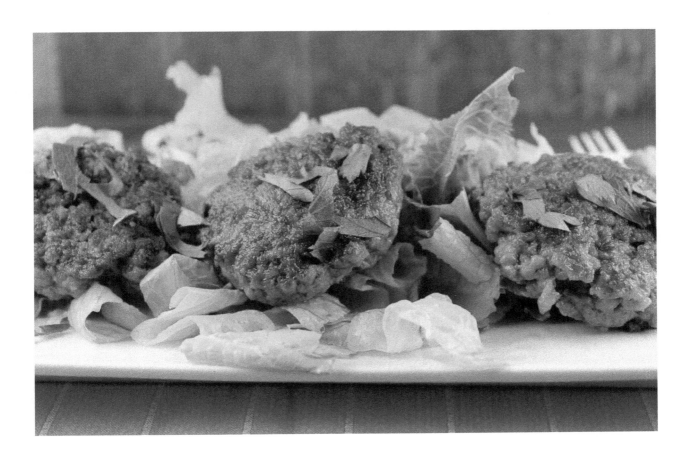

# SALMON STUFFED AVOCADOS

Mini avocados make perfect appetizers or snacks when stuffed with savory ingredients like salmon and veggies.

MAKES 4 SERVING/ TOTAL TIME 10 MINUTE

## INGREDIENTS

6 oz can wild caught salmon drained

1/4 cup onion diced

2 tablespoon minced pimentos

1 tablespoon olive oil

1 tablespoon chopped fresh parsley

Juice of 1 lemon

2 mini avocados

## METHOD

**STEP 1**

Combine the salmon, onion, pimentos, olive oil, parsley, and lemon juice in a small bowl. Mix well.

When ready to serve, cut the avocados in half and remove the pit. Fill the avocado halves with the salmon mixture right before serving.

**NUTRITION  VALUE**

200 Kcal, 10g fat,
10g fiber, 20g protein, 15g carbs.

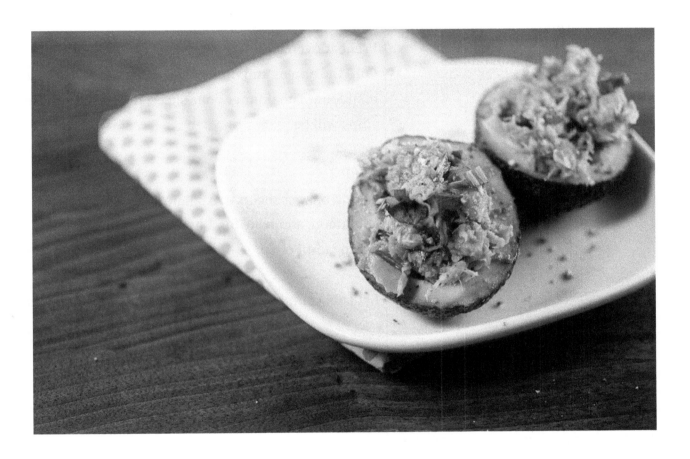

# OVEN APPLE CHIPS

If you're looking for something crispy, healthy, and flavorful, these apple chips will hit the spot. They're easy to make, don't require any special equipment, and are super addicting. Use your favorite kind of apple, or a mix.

MAKES 4 SERVING/ TOTAL TIME 2 HOUR

## INGREDIENTS

4 apples any kind

1 teaspoon ground cinnamon

## METHOD

### STEP 1

Preheat oven to 200 degrees F.

Core the apples and thinly slice using a sharp knife or mandolin. The thinner your slices, the crispier the apple chips will be.

### STEP 2

Lay on baking sheets in a single layer, sprinkle on cinnamon, and bake for 1 hour. Flip, and continue baking until crisp.

Let cool completely, and store in an airtight container.

## NUTRITION  VALUE

354 Kcal, 17g fat,
10g fiber, 33g protein, 14g carbs.

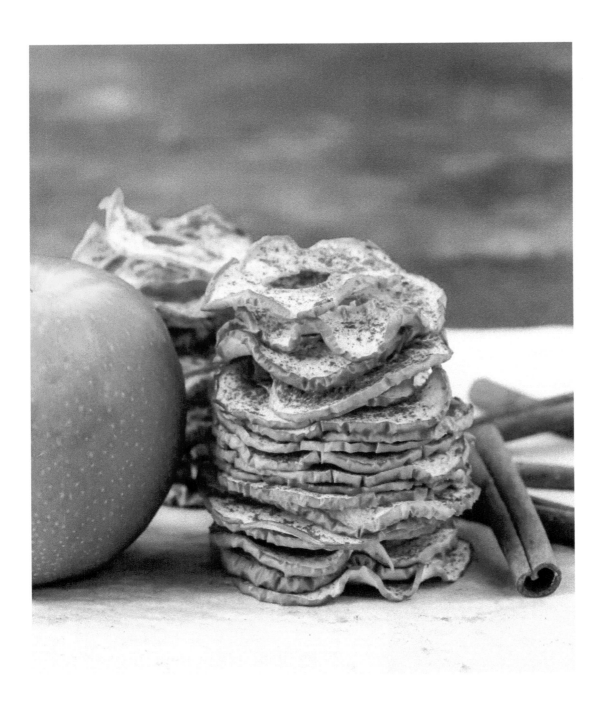

# FRESH SUMMER SALSA

When fresh tomatoes abound, salsa is the perfect party food. It's quick, flavorful, and easy to customize. This makes a good Paleo party food when served with crunchy veggies, but it's also a great topper for grilled chicken or fish.

MAKES 1 SERVING/ TOTAL TIME 10 MINUTE

## INGREDIENTS

4 large tomatoes diced

1 green bell pepper diced

1 red onion diced

1 small bunch cilantro chopped

2 cloves garlic minced

1 teaspoon ground cumin

Juice of 2 limes

1 tablespoon avocado or olive oil

Sea salt and fresh ground pepper to taste

## METHOD

**STEP 1**

Combine all of the ingredients in a large bowl and toss until well combined. Refrigerate until ready to serve to allow the flavors to meld.

**NUTRITION  VALUE**

335 Kcal, 14g fat,
8g fiber, 32g protein, 15g carbs.

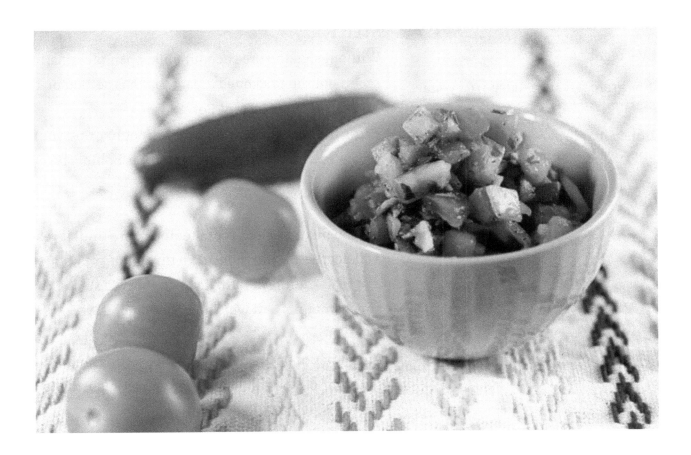

# COCONUT YOGURT

This is one of the recipes using your Instant Pot that isn't exactly instant, but it is worth the trouble.

MAKES 8 SERVING/ TOTAL TIME 3 HOUR

## INGREDIENTS

3 cans coconut milk refrigerated overnight

1 5- gram package dairy-free yogurt starter

Honey maple syrup, or other Paleo-approved sweetener, optional

## METHOD

**STEP 1**

Without shaking the coconut milk, open the cans, and scoop out the thickened cream that has settled on top. Add this to your Instant Pot.

Press the "yogurt" setting on your pot to bring your cream to a boil. When your mixture is boiling, turn off your pot.

**STEP 2**

Let the mixture sit at room temperature until it reaches 100 degrees F, and then add a tiny bit of your starter, and whisk until smooth. Keep adding the starter in small amounts and whisking until smooth.

**STEP 3**

Turn the pot back on to the yogurt setting, and set the timer for 6-8 hours. The longer you let it go, the tangier the flavor will be.

**STEP 4**

When done, whisk in honey or maple syrup to taste. Transfer to an airtight container and refrigerate for 6-8 hours, until thick and creamy.

**NUTRITION  VALUE**

335 Kcal, 14g fat, 8g fiber, 32g protein, 15g carbs.

Unbelievable Paleo   Jamie Evans

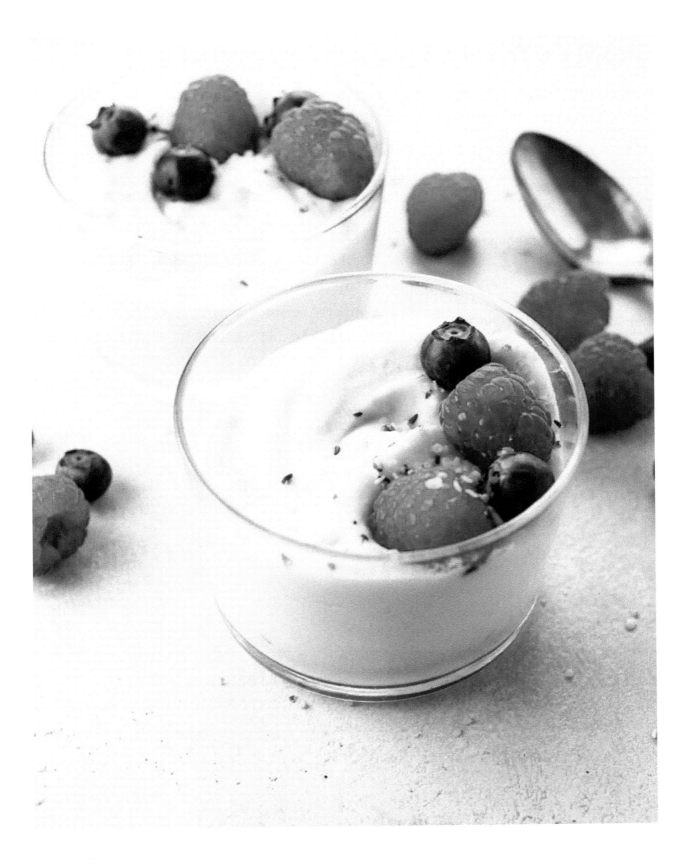

# POMEGRANATE CABBAGE SALAD

This winter salad is crisp, bright, and delicious, and perfect as a hearty side dish. The bright tangy dressing brings it all together and makes it shine.

MAKES 4 SERVING/ TOTAL TIME 20 MINUTE

## INGREDIENTS

4 cups shredded cabbage red, green, or mixture

1 shredded carrot

1/4 cup chopped parsley

1/2 cup pomegranate arils

1/2 cup olive oil

3 tablespoons white wine vinegar

1 teaspoon Dijon mustard

1 teaspoon maple syrup or pomegranate molasses

Sea salt and fresh ground pepper to taste

## METHOD

**STEP 1**

Put the cabbage, carrots, parsley, and pomegranate arils in large bowl and toss well.

Whisk the remaining ingredients in a small bowl or shake in a jar and toss with the salad before serving.

## NUTRITION VALUE

625 Kcal, 20 fat,
11g fiber, 54.2g protein, 14 carbs.

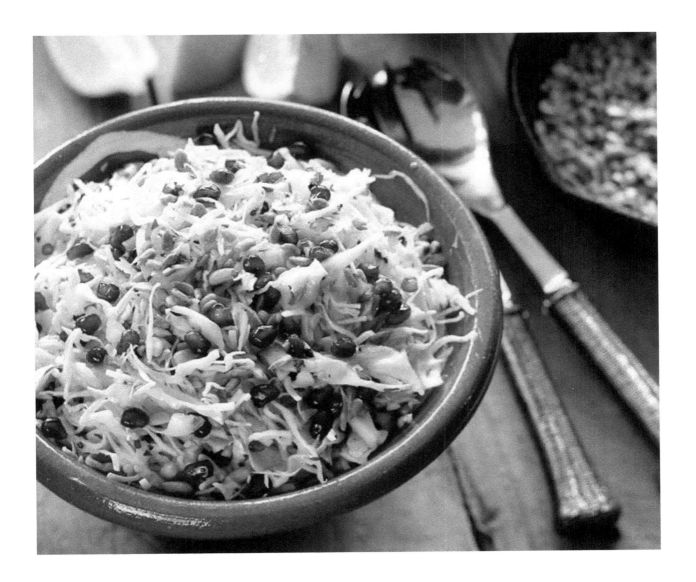

Lightning Source UK Ltd.
Milton Keynes UK
UKHW050634010621
384724UK00003B/6